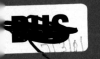

Healing Plants

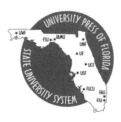

Florida A&M University, Tallahassee
Florida Atlantic University, Boca Raton
Florida Gulf Coast University, Ft. Myers
Florida International University, Miami
Florida State University, Tallahassee
University of Central Florida, Orlando
University of Florida, Gainesville
University of North Florida, Jacksonville
University of South Florida, Tampa
University of West Florida, Pensacola

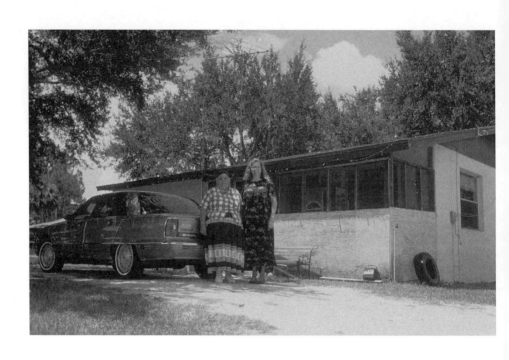

Healing Plants

Medicine of the Florida Seminole Indians

Alice Micco Snow and Susan Enns Stans

University Press of Florida

Gainesville · Tallahassee · Tampa · Boca Raton

Pensacola · Orlando · Miami · Jacksonville · Ft. Myers

06 05 04 03 02 01 6 5 4 3 2 1

Publication of this book was supported in part by a grant
from the Seminole Tribe of Florida.

Library of Congress Cataloging-in-Publication Data

Snow, Alice Micco, 1922–
Healing plants: medicine of the Florida Seminole Indians /
Alice Micco Snow and Susan Enns Stans.
p. cm.
Includes bibliographical references and index.
ISBN 0-8130-2062-X (cloth: acid-free paper)
1. Seminole Indians—Ethnobotany. 2. Seminole Indians—Medicine.
3. Medicinal plants—Florida. I. Stans, Susan Enns, 1942–. II. Title.
E99.S28 S66 2001
615'.32'089973—dc21 00-069078

The University Press of Florida is the scholarly publishing agency
for the State University System of Florida, comprising Florida A&M
University, Florida Atlantic University, Florida Gulf Coast Univer-
sity, Florida International University, Florida State University, Uni-
versity of Central Florida, University of Florida, University of
North Florida, University of South Florida, and University of West
Florida.

University Press of Florida
15 Northwest 15th Street
Gainesville, FL 32611–2079
http://www.upf.com

Contents

The color section "Plants and Their Properties" follows page 80

Photographs

Color Plates

1. Akkotorkv (lotus)
2. Akwanv (willow)
3. Cafaknv (huckleberry, blueberry)
4. Culoswuce (little muscadine grape or southern fox grape)
5. Cule (slash pine)
6. Este lopockuce emeto ("where the little people live")
7. Eto-hvtkv (Carolina ash)
8. Heles-here ("the good medicine," downy milk pea)
9. Heles-hvtke (ginseng)
10. Helokhakv (rubber plant, strangler fig)
11. Heno (red maple)
12. Hetotvpe (frost weed)
13. Kowike entvlako (quail's foot, partridge pea, or bird's foot trefoil)
14. Kvfockv (penny royal sage, peppermint)
15. Kvnrvkko (prickly pear)
16. Kvsvkakuce (rattle box, rabbit bells)
17. Lucv-huehkv enhompetv (gopher turtle food, gopher apple)
18. Opv 'mvhoswv (mallow)
19. Passv (button snakeroot)
20. Pvrko (grape)
21. Roheleko (mistletoe)
22. 'Stvlokpuce (beggar's lice)
23. 'Stvlokpuce hvlwat (beggar's lice)
24. Svpeyv (small one, candy root, polygala)
25. Svpeyv rakko (big one, lantana)
26. Tolv (red bay)
27. Torkop-rakko (water hemlock)
28. Tvwv (winged sumac)
29. Ue-heleswv (lizard's tail)
30. Vcenv (cedar)
31. Wēso (sassafras)
32. Wotko empvrko (raccoon grapes)
33. Yvnvsv heleswv (black root)

Forewords

In every profession there is usually an assistant. Doctors, lawyers, and Indian chiefs have assistants. And so it is that Seminole medicine men and women call upon people who have a special knowledge of certain plants, roots, barks, and other items that need to be collected for the medicine they make. Every ailment or sickness, be it physical or psychological, has different formulas for curing. The medicine men and women give the prayers, chant, and prepare the medicine for usage or application. Alice Snow belongs to the very special small group of people who have this knowledge. It is with honor that I have known and worked with Alice for many years and have seen how her endeavor to pass her knowledge to others will continue through the generations.

Sho·naa·bish

Ah·ne

> James E. Billie, chairman,
> *Seminole Tribe of Florida*

◆ ◆ ◆

I have known Alice all my life. I remember Alice and Mama at home in the camp. They would go out and work every day to provide for the family and then have dinner for us—even though they worked all day long. Mama [Leona Micco Smith] and Alice would leave the house about six o'clock, while it was still dark, to make sure they got there on time. They picked tomatoes or worked in the field or planted grass. After a field had been disked, they picked up palmetto roots and piled them up so they could be burned to clear a field. Alice said they would sometimes find medicine under the ground after it was disked and save it for later. We kids would tag along either to get in the way or to help. I might look after my younger brother and sister, trying to keep them from getting into trouble.

I was around the medicine all the time. My mother would get medicine for us all the time. We were all in one camp and we would use the same medicine. Me and my brother or whoever was sick would take it. I remember drinking the medicine and using it all over. I remember having an earache, and Mama would take me to someone who would sing and blow in my ear to cure it. I didn't know what was going on. Someone would tell us how to use the medicine, and that was it. We were only playing around. We had no realization about what we had. Just someone in the family got it, and we all had to use the medicine. It wasn't until we were grown that we knew what it was. It was just part of our lives. Now we know when we use outside medicine, because we have to drive to the doctor.

My mother was always there when you needed her. She was always using Indian medicine for sickness. She and Alice would know who would treat the medicine with songs. They even started going to Oklahoma and using their medicine and doctors there. They went to different people, not only different places where they knew people who knew medicine. Alice said when Mama went to look for medicine, she would want her to go along. Alice sometimes called the doctors on the phone when Mama wanted the medicine treated or sometimes took the medicine to be exchanged.

I remember that when I started working with the Tribe's program to help alcoholics, Alice was already there trying to get people on the medicine [vwotickv or "on the wagon" medicine] and working with other agencies to send them to treatment if they didn't want to use the Indian medicine. She still works with the medicine today, but as an employee of the Tribe, teaching anyone who is interested. One day when she was working for her medicine program, she was writing up the Indian words in the office. I would see her write them down, the Creek word names, just like she said them. She would say each word and write it just like it sounded.

People learn the medicine by being around it. Today, Alice is still teaching her daughter Salina about the medicine by being around her. Our kids would learn it by being around Mama, Rosie Billie (my cousin), or Alice. We are still doing that today. We still use it, and it works. You have to collect medicine to get to know it. For four or five years, Alice has been teaching her son Elbert about collecting, and after a while he learned this skill. Alice might die next year, and we wouldn't know the medicine she knows. With her book, at least we will know what kind of medicine to use.

It is important for our youth to learn about the medicine. Today our kids are going to public school and have lost most of our language. Our parents told us to go to school because we were coming into the big world and we needed it to survive. Now our children don't know the language and don't know that way of life.

Other things don't help keep the language. My wife, Lois, speaks Mikasuki, and I speak Creek, and my kids don't speak either. They don't know the use of the medicine—they will use it when told to, but we have to remind them what is going on. Lois will get the medicine and give it to them when they need it, like my mom did. If they knew about the medicine, it would be here in the future.

When someone dies, we use the medicine. The only time we can teach the medicine is during the four days after the death. Someone has to collect the medicine after a death and have an Indian doctor treat it. Only a few people treat the medicine now, and we might lose it. With this book we can learn all the herbs, and that is what Alice has been teaching her son and daughter.

Jack Smith, Jr.
Brighton Council representative for the Seminole Tribe of Florida

◆ ◆ ◆

My mother, Alice Snow, has been the most influential person in my life from the moment of my birth. Reflecting on the past, I remember that Mom would always make it a point to teach us something every day. She constantly told us, "Be proud of our Indian heritage and cultural customs, especially the Indian medicine."

When I was about five or six years old, my mother told me she was going to teach me to be an Indian doctor for earache pains. I asked her, "Don't you think I'm too young?" and she said, "No." I then asked, "Why me? Can't you teach one of the others?" and she told me, "No" again. Before I could ask my next question, she explained the following: "From one generation to the next generation, the knowledge is usually passed on through the youngest child. And if I teach you now, you will always remember the words." (And guess what? I still do.) Remembering my first patient, an elderly man, I laughed when he told me he had an earache, and he wanted me to doctor it for him. I told him, "My mom can do it. I'll get her," but he said, "You are the doctor now."

As I got older, my mother taught me how to make medicine for someone who has suffered from a bad cut or wound and for sharp pains in the stomach. During the process of doing these Indian medicines, I speak or sing in the Seminole language, which I cannot translate into English to understand. All I know is I carry this small portion of our Indian tradition with great pride, and someday it will be up to me to pass on the knowledge to the next generation.

Over the past few years, my mother has been guiding my brother, Elbert, in the direction of looking for medicine plants and herbs. There's a lot out there to learn, and time is running short for our elders, who have the knowledge of our Seminole Indian medicine traits.

I am very, very proud of my mother, who has taken the time to do research for this book. All her hard work will be appreciated for many years to come and may serve as one of the greatest accomplishments in Seminole medicine.

In every child's life there should always be a mentor, who is responsible for preserving the past, nurturing the present, and preparing us for the future. For me, that's my mom, Alice Snow, and I love her dearly.

Salina N. Dorgan,
Alice's daughter

Acknowledgments

I am writing this book because young people need to learn Indian medicine before it is lost. White medicine will not cure all of the sicknesses, so it is important that my people have the knowledge to carry on a long tradition of healing.

I learned Indian medicine from my mother, Emma Micco. I went with her into the woods to collect the herbs. She would tell me what each plant was used for and what to call it in Creek. I learned some of my information from Indian doctors, Josie Billie, Jimmie Tommie, Buffalo Jim, Sonny Billie, Pete Osceola, Frank Shore, Rosie Billie, Bobby Billie, Susie Billie, Tony Billie, Louise Doctor, Joe Doctor, and my father, Charlie Micco. They were the ones who told me what plants to get for the treatment of the people. I want to thank them and Jack Smith, Jr., James E. Billie, and Michelle Thomas for their support.

As I got older, I found out the Mikasuki and English names. In this book, I have provided the three different names to the best of my ability. Different people have different pronunciations and items for treatment, but the ones in this book are recorded as I learned them.

The Indian doctor tells the gatherers of medicine what to bring to him. The preparations included in this book must be treated with the Indian doctor's songs in order for them to be effective. This book tells only what the herbs are and what I was told to gather for each of the treatments. Some people think the medicine shouldn't be shared with outsiders, but these are just names of plants. It used to be a secret, a long time ago, but it's not now. We even treat *este-lvste* and *este-hvtke* now.

Another person who was important to me and my knowledge of the herbs was my sister, Leona Smith, who died in 1999. She was always helping me find some of the plants. I also thank Susan Stans for preparing my handwritten notes to make this book. Norman Tribbett, Jack Martin, Mary Frances Johns, Mary C. Johns, Betty Cypress, and Minnie Micco helped me, too.

Mvto,
Alice Snow

A Cherished Tradition

♦♦♦♦♦♦♦♦♦♦♦♦♦♦♦♦♦♦♦

Alice Snow is both a traditional Seminole Native American and a cultural innovator who combines the old ways with new methods of preserving and teaching "Indian medicine" (*heleswv*). This book came about because Alice recognized that fewer and fewer people in the Seminole Tribe were using traditional medicine and fewer still collected or knew the songs to treat the herbs, thus providing the herbs with healing power. She began by carefully writing down individual treatments on a yellow legal pad that she kept in her closet. Now she and I have collaborated on a book that describes the treatments she has made for Indian doctors' cures and defines the taxonomy of plants she collects. Alice is not an Indian doctor herself but is an important link between the doctor and the patient. Because she provides raw material or herb medicine for treatment, she is somewhat like a modern pharmacist. This book is a result of three years of apprenticeship, discussion, and fieldwork at Brighton Reservation near Okeechobee in South Florida.

Part I presents a picture of the Seminole history, native medicine, and Alice's life to illuminate the indigenous healing practices in cultural context and to provide background for part II—the herbal handbook—a guide for tribal members to become collectors themselves. By putting her knowledge in print, Alice gives future generations the means to learn to identify and collect the material if the "Indian doctors" are gone and the language is lost. Traditional styles of learning are difficult to maintain when circumscribed by a separate and intrusive majority culture. As a people greatly disrupted by the invasion of European settlers and still suspicious of "outsiders" (*este ētv fullat*),[1] many Seminoles will criticize Alice for revealing some secrets of the medicine to the world through print. Alice is willing to withstand that criticism to preserve her teachings for her children, grandchildren, and great-grandchildren and to make a reference book for all tribal members. She feels comfortable in describing the medicine collection process. The real secrets are in the songs the Indian doctor uses to empower the treatment with healing properties.

We hope that biomedical practitioners will read the book to capture the essence of Seminole medicine and its core belief so that they can more effectively treat their Seminole patients. We further hope the biomedical practitioners will honor and respect the age-old practices, which are used not as a substitute for Western healing techniques but as a supplement. Although its focus is the Seminole people, the book offers any nontribal reader a glimpse into a primary belief system so as to foster understanding between two diverse cultural groups.

Herbal medicine is linked closely to the oral tradition. It has been passed down from generation to generation, from parent to child—what anthropologists call enculturation—learned through the imitation and reproduction of cultural behavior. Western medicine has been available to the tribe since before its formation in 1957; the Seminole medicine persists as local wisdom in a network of Indian doctors and collectors in the various Florida Seminole communities. Although community members fear losing their culture and language, unwritten knowledge tends to persist in small communities and particularly those in semi-isolation from the majority culture. Seminole medicine continues to be practiced in Alice's community, not because of its quaintness as a custom of old but as a cherished tradition. Because of this persistence in use, it has a special place alongside Western medicine. Western medicine instills a belief in cure through drugs, pills, or prophylactics, but not all ailments attended by Western physicians are 100 percent affected. As a result, Seminole medicine is useful in treating the chronic symptoms, the psychological aspects of disease, and even the side effects of Western medication. It may be a community member's first response to illness or the last resort when biomedical treatments fail to cure the individual. The book is not meant to replace the oral tradition but to enhance it. The treatments should not be looked upon as the definitive ingredients for a cure, but rather they represent the herbs collected relating to a particular Indian doctor's request at one point in time.

In 1993, I first visited the Brighton Reservation to gain permission to conduct my dissertation research there. Anthropology is grounded in long-term studies—living in a community using ethnographic methods and describing a group's beliefs, attitudes, and behaviors. I had grown up in a neighboring county but still knew little about the Seminoles at Brighton. I wanted to know more and to build a bridge of understanding between my world and our native Florida people. I met with Jack Smith, Jr., the Brighton Council representative, to get permission. He stated that it was not up to him to grant permission but up to the individuals themselves to volunteer to answer questions. I needed a place to stay, so he suggested his aunt, Alice Snow, who was a tribal elder living alone in a three-bedroom house. After meeting me, she agreed that I could stay with her. She liked having the company, and I could help her clean and cook.

When I first came to live with Alice, she was asked to prepare medicine for her son-in-law's mother. Alice asked me to come along. After a day of collecting herbs and taking notes to record the process, she told me she had begun a book. She took it out of the closet when I asked if I could see it. The manuscript impressed me, and I offered to help her prepare it for publication.

I asked Alice to explain many of the techniques and nuances involved in Seminole medicine. She knew the material so well that she was not aware of the knowledge behind her knowledge. I continually asked why, what else, and how, to make the book as comprehensive as possible. Alice described the herbs, what the derivative plants look like, where they are found, and how they are used.

Alice and I went to the University of Florida Herbarium to identify the botanical names of the less common plants. We sketched plants, involving her grandson Jay Holata and a young Seminole woman, Tommie Motlow Micco, in drawing some of the herbs. Finally, Alice began drawing the herbs herself. We have included the pencil and pen-and-ink drawings among her treatments. Most of the drawings are of herbs, which she recognizes as medicinal, but their use in specific medicines has been lost. They are identified by their Creek names because in some instances their botanical names have not been found.

Initially, we planned to provide a desktop copy from my computer. As the first draft evolved, others in the tribe showed an interest. Alice's nephew Jack Smith, Jr., was one of those people. In fact, he had frequently encouraged her to write the book. Then Michelle Thomas, the tribal chairman's assistant, became interested, so Alice showed the preliminary pages to James Billie, the tribal chairman. Shortly thereafter, tribal funds were set aside for Alice's expenses to continue her project. We continued to collaborate from then on. She provided the raw knowledge, and I recorded, photographed, and edited the manuscript.

Alice Snow is truly bicultural—a term used by anthropologists to describe people who negotiate their daily life from one culture to another, incorporating the best parts of each culture into the other and knowing the rules of social behavior in each. Alice recognizes the influence European-American-style education has on her people and has adopted both a Western style and traditional ways of teaching native healing. Western education has brought a shift in traditional learning, from imitation, stories, and lessons from the elders to becoming literate in English, relying on books, media, and the school system to identify important knowledge.

Language

Alice knows Creek and most Mikasuki names for medicinal herbs and other useful plants. If a plant has no known use as medicine or food, or has been recently introduced, she generally does not have a Creek name for it. If a plant has been introduced since the use of English in schools, the plant with no antiquity will have an English common name. The fact that some Creek names for herbs are so similar to the common English names leads me to believe that the Seminole ancestors introduced these herbs to settlers. Creek nouns are literal descriptors for some plants, for instance, *lucvhuehkv enhompetv* means "gopher turtle food" (referring to its fruit), and its common name is gopher apple. No medicine that Alice has told me about has an English name only.

Early anthropologists Franz Boas and Paul Radin wrote about the importance of native informants writing about their own culture. My collaboration with Alice on this book was also intended to foster indigenous authorship, inspired by the work of H. Russell Bernard and Jesus Salinas Pedraza in their book *Native Ethnography* (1989).[2] Bernard and Salinas Pedraza promote the native informant writing in his or her own language with a modified computer keyboard, but Alice and I have included only a portion of the Creek and Mikasuki words and no native language prose at all.[3]

Certainly the most important part of using the language involves the plant names. Without those, the usefulness of the book to tribal members is questionable. We have used the alphabet from Oklahoma that is taught in the university there (see appendix B). Margaret Mauldin, a Creek teacher and fluent Creek writer, and Jack Martin, linguist at the College of William and Mary, have helped us write the Creek and Mikasuki words in a more standardized spelling. No one among the Florida Seminoles writes with native fluency. Alice's and my phonetic spelling of the herbs is shown at the end of the book for reading novices in Creek and Mikasuki (see appendix A). Much of the text is taken from Alice's own words in English and conveys a sense of how she sees the world.

When I met Alice she had already begun her book. She had carefully written about six treatments on a worn yellow legal pad. She had many items that were simply abbreviated, such as "c." I had to ask her to fill in the blank, which she readily did from memory. Although I wrote from Alice's own written notes many times, I used the "as told to" method to clarify details of her treatments. I tried not only to retain the original flavor of Alice's words but also to solicit additional information. I changed Alice's English to clarify the prose; for example, I added referents that are configured differently in her native language, Creek. By reading the edited works back, we were able to negotiate meaning. I even attempted to write some of the treatments in Creek.

A book about Seminole treatments and herbs serves two main functions of writing.[4] First, writing serves to store knowledge, allowing ideas to be communicated over time and space. It marks and records language (mnemonics) as it is spoken at the time and permits the second function of writing—deciphering the grammar. Although tape recordings also store knowledge, only writing functions to provide a visual domain in which to examine language. In writing, one can inspect the ordering and reordering of words and sentences. Writing facilitates the process of reorganization and permanently affects oral communication. Not only does it change the nature of verbal communication by adding to it, but it exists even after the natural spoken language has disappeared. Written language preserves material that is rarely used in ordinary speech. This is not to place a higher value on written language over spoken language but to offer a different aspect of language, one that offers another method of learning—visualization.

Anthropologists today are ethically bound to return to the community the information they gather. The vehicles for doing so are varied. As an anthropologist, I supported Alice's efforts by helping her organize her oral communications, identifying the herbs by common and Latin names, and giving technical assistance in assembling the book. This book records the oral history as seen by one woman, Alice Snow. It focuses on gathering and assembling medicine as she has experienced it. I incorporated other facets of Alice's life—a lifestyle that is rapidly disappearing for Native Americans as they become more and more acculturated through contact with their white neighbors, adopt new technology, and are educated in local public schools in the Western traditions.

Experiences with Alice in the Field

Recording Alice's knowledge required that I experience all aspects of herb collection. We began quite unexpectedly. Our first excursion began early one morning in the spring of 1995, when Alice said, "Come with me." She assembled an ax, a long-bladed steel knife, and a brown grocery bag, and we were off to comb the countryside for Indian medicine. Alice drove that first time. As she drove us along the main road leading to the Brighton Seminole Reservation, she stared into the green thickets to the left and right. She came to a spot where the roadside was meshed with greenery, slowing to a crawl. Then, unexpectedly, she put the car into reverse and maneuvered back down the road. She pulled onto the shoulder on the left side, stopped, and said, "Go get that."

"What?" I replied.

"The *tolv* over there."

I looked—perplexed—into a verdant mass of bushes, trees, and undergrowth, seeing only green. I got out of the car and moved in the direction Alice had pointed. "This?" I questioned, pointing to each different plant and asking repeatedly until she nodded her head. I broke off a few leaves and took them to her. "That's it," she said.

She had seen the bay tree (*Persea borbonia*) easily among the roadside array, and I had seen only green. At the time, I had no idea about Indian medicine, but I was becoming Alice's legs and, later, her driver for her forays into the woods.

When I met Alice, she was a vital seventy-two-year-old who seemed to have boundless energy. She recognized the limits of her activities in the woods, having had two knee replacements in the previous two years. At Alice's age she was willing to have a younger person traipse through canals and high weeds for the treasured herbs. I was fascinated and more than willing to help someone who had given a needy graduate student a home while she did her dissertation research in the community in exchange for housekeeping and cooking. The housekeeping and cooking were to become a private joke between us later when, finding myself exhausted from my ethnographic work, I would suggest that we forget the house and go out to dinner. I persisted in my role of driver, offering to get myself a chauffeur's cap. I spent time jumping canals, climbing over barbed wire fences, and wading into swampy areas to retrieve the herbs she had spotted. She remained strategically positioned in her car so she could clearly see to point out the needed plants. At times, she gave up in exasperation at my inability to see a particular item that I had no knowledge of, and she, too, entered into the wet. I would bring back samples to the car for her approval and to receive instructions to get more or throw away the excess. The amount was tailored to the particular patient's need. When she collected the bark from the willow, it was particularly important to gauge the amount by knowledge of the intended recipient. A white person would need less because medicine strong enough for an Indian would be too strong for a white person's constitution. Alice believes that many of the treatments are too strong for *este-hvtke*, or "white people," and may cause harm if caution is not used.

While she waited in the car, Alice would sometimes cut the herbs into smaller pieces to fit into the grocery bag. After collecting an array of herbs, we would head back to her home to complete the process. At home she would cut up the herbs into even smaller pieces in order to fit them into a plastic gallon milk container, then pour water into the container until it was three-quarters full. After the concoction was prepared, Alice would set out to find the doctor. Sometimes she called ahead to find out where to meet him or her, and other times she would just drive to the doctor's house to take the mix of herbs. Once we waited in the living room of a doctor's house while he removed himself and the jug to a back room to "fix" the medicine (*heleswv vkpofketv*). To do this, the Indian doctor would blow air into the water in the jug with a straw and sing a repetitive song over the mixture. He would alternate these actions. Another time we met Sonny Billie, a noted Miccosukee doctor, in an orange grove where he was operating a front-end loader as part of his regular job. We agreed to meet him later at the senior "hot meals" building. He received the herbs from us, moved to a small chickee on the side of the building, and sang and blew into the medicine to treat it as we waited in the car.

Generally, the treatment takes a half hour or more. When the treatment was especially long, we would leave and come back later. One of the reasons native medicine knowledge is dying out is that it takes apprentices an inordinate amount of time to memorize the songs that are learned aurally rather than reinforced through reading. Several younger people have at times met with older doctors for a number of days to learn the words. Many of the mothers know a few of the shorter songs, like the ones for earaches, since they are easier to learn. These mothers will treat their children or kin without taking them to the Indian doctor, having learned the chant from a medicine man, much as Alice learned the song from her father.

Finding the correct herb to collect was only the first part of my learning experience. I learned traditional ways of teaching—observing and doing. I wandered into swampy, muddy areas to collect *ue-heleswv*, across canals to collect *akwanv* bark—even over fences and up trees. Sometimes we drove as many as thirty miles to find a special herb. Alice could always pick out the herb while riding by in the car. I felt much better when I began driving and she began seeking the right plant from the passenger seat of the car. Sometimes she would locate a spot where a particular herb grew, and we would return to that spot for that herb over and over. Sometimes she had only in mind what grew with what. *Tolv* could be found growing above the saw palmettos (*Serenoa repens*). *Roheleko* was found in oak trees. *Lucvhuehkv enhompetv* could be found in high sandy areas. The landscape began to change for me. Instead of a repetitive green, I began to see relationships between plants, how Alice organized her gathering, and medicine everywhere. Traditionalists use herbs from the world around us—we have only to look.

Alice's Effort to Preserve the Medicine

The two native languages, Mikasuki and Muskogee/Creek, are in danger of being lost. Because of intermarriage, because English is used as the lingua franca within the tribe, and because English has been accorded higher prestige through the educational system, the Seminoles are in a difficult position. They recognize the need to be proficient in English to cope with the outside world and the need to preserve their own language to maintain the culture's unique healing system. Yet it is not through books that people are immersed in the stream of spoken knowledge that flows through their communities.[5] With the loss of language and the shift to medicalization of community health, Alice decided to provide her community with an opportunity to learn the traditional medicine in the format they had become accustomed to through public education. Alice spoke to a youth conference about the services she offers as part of her Indian medicine program for the tribe: "I am starting a program for one year, an Indian medicine training program. I am going to go around and tell those Indian people, 'If somebody wants to use the Indian medicine, they can come to me and I will get the medicine. I have the material. As long as the money [from the tribal council's funding] holds out.' I want to tell them the culture I was talking about. That's why I want you to pick it up. I am going to get an Indian doctor and they can teach you the songs. And learn the treatment. When you get married, you can get a treatment to keep you from separating. Even when ya'll are having babies, you can treat them with Indian medicine. Some Christians say not to use it, but *Hesaketvmesē* [God or Breathmaker] put it there for us to use."

As part of her mission to pass on the knowledge of herb collecting and the procedures, Alice and I dedicate this book to the Seminole people. May their traditions continue.

I

Background

1

The Seminole People

♦♦♦♦♦♦♦♦♦♦♦♦♦♦♦♦♦♦

A complete understanding of traditional medicine begins with an overview of the Seminole people—their history and traditional practices and their political incorporation and transformation today. The historical displacement of the people from one environment to another changed the medicine available. Their adjustment to the majority American culture transformed their social patterns endangering their centuries-old healing practices.

History

The Seminoles are an amalgamation of Native American groups from the Upper and Lower Creek confederation from Georgia and Alabama who were pushed into Florida as early as the 1700s by the encroachment of white settlers into the South. They formerly lived in towns, which featured higher population densities, farming, and wattle and daub homes located along waterways. They moved into Timucuan, Calusa, and other tribal lands decimated by diseases brought to the New World by the explorers. The first to arrive were the Hitchiti-speaking group, later to become the Mikasuki language speakers. Eventually the Upper Creek or Muskogee/ Creek-speaking groups followed. Smaller portions of other distinct language groups were to blend into the Miccosukee and Creek communities.

Not recognizing the distinctive differences in languages that designated the separate groups, settlers and soldiers attached their own name for the amalgamation of groups. Their new name became Seminole, from the Mikasuki (the linguistic spelling of the language) and Creek word *semvnole*,[1] which means "undomesticated" or "untamed," but ultimately from the Spanish word *cimarrón*, which means "wild" or "runaway."[2] On the surface, they appeared to be one cultural group because of the shared aspects of their daily lives. However, the people themselves understood the distinctiveness of the separate groups in their mutually unintelligible languages. Later, runaway slaves established towns and shared traditions with the earlier groups in Spanish Florida. They were to become known as the Black Seminoles.[3]

For a while, the Seminoles were able to carve more permanent communities in Florida, planting fields of corn. This was not to last, as the new American colonies were to spread their domain into Spanish Florida. The First Seminole War occurred in 1817–18 and ended in Andrew Jackson's raid against Spanish territory in Florida. Again, the war forced the breakup of towns and pushed the Seminoles farther south. The Spanish gave up control of Florida to the United States in 1821. In 1823, the Treaty of Moultrie Creek limited the Seminoles to a large parcel of less desirable land in Central Florida. The Seminoles were not pleased with the arrangement. In just ten years, new pressures from settlers into Florida caused the government to attempt to remove the Seminoles to Oklahoma. Some, not wanting further bloodshed, agreed to relocate. Others would neither move nor return Seminole slaves who had joined them for protection, and further skirmishes ensued. Osceola was to lead them.

During the Second Seminole War, 1835–42, most of the Seminoles, including Osceola, who later died in prison, were captured. About 1,600 U.S. troops and civilians were lost, along with much matériel, costing the government an estimated $30 to $40 million.[4] Seminole fatalities numbered in the hundreds. As many as 4,000 or more captured Seminole and black men, women, and children were forcibly transported to lands in Oklahoma, leaving possibly only 400 in Florida, most of them Mikasuki speakers. The remaining groups scattered into the wilderness of the southernmost portions of Florida, forming small mobile camps of related kin. Their flight from settlers and soldiers was a successful tactic in avoiding deportation or death, until the Third, and final, Seminole War of 1855–57, which led to the capture and exile of Billy Bowlegs and his group. The remaining groups were estimated to number between 150 and 200 Seminoles, from which the present-day population is descended.

Each consecutive disruption pushed the people farther and farther into South Florida. By disappearing into the Everglades, they were protected from the U.S. military and deportation to Oklahoma, but this strategy, while making survival possible, disrupted earlier subsistence patterns of farming supplemented with wild game. In South Florida, the Seminoles became increasingly dependent upon hunting and gathering to feed their families. Crops would have to be hidden far from their small encampments, lest they reveal their location to the soldiers. Soldiers, hoping to flush out the elusive Seminoles, relied on destruction of crops to force them out of hiding.

More and more, the Seminoles relied on gathered material, such as coontie, palmetto berries, other wild plants, and game, for their daily sustenance. Their complex villages became things of the past. Each family utilized available materials to construct their family encampment, located on high ground in the watery everglades or tucked away in a hardwood hammock. The open-air, palmetto-thatched roofs of their chickees—*chickee* is the Mikasuki word for "house"—became the distinctive feature of their habitation areas and later a symbol of their very Indianness. Seminoles continued to live in scattered camps into the first half of the twentieth century.

The Seminole Tribe Today

The Seminoles living in a loose association of camps throughout South Florida incorporated into a formal political entity in 1956. Since then, the Tribe's leaders have focused on establishing self-reliance through economic programs and education.[5] Their subsistence practices have changed from hunting and gathering to joining the wage labor market, and the Tribe has instituted programs to provide its members with a way of making a living. In the 1930s, a cattle program was established that still offers employment and individual cattle ownership. Other programs include citrus and vegetable farming, gaming in the form of high-stakes bingo, and tobacco sales. Profits from these main ventures support the Tribe's infrastructure and provide employment, educational, and social benefits to tribal members. The group also holds food and craft festivals that attract visitors and contribute to the members' income. The Tribe employs a majority of members, either in one of its business enterprises or as part of Bureau of Indian Affairs programs.

Today, the Seminole Tribe of Florida[6] is a federally recognized, political and economic entity of approximately 2,500 Native Americans who mainly inhabit the six reservations in South Florida: the Hollywood, Brighton, Big Cypress, Tampa, Immokalee, and Fort Pierce locations.[7] Although all communities share a rich cultural tradition, the people mostly speak two distinct Native languages within the organization, in addition to English. The languages, Mikasuki and Creek/Muskogee, are related but mutually unintelligible. Many of the younger persons speak English only, and a decreasing portion of the people are bilingual or trilingual.

The Tribe consists of eight matrilineal clans around which reciprocal relations and affiliations are based. Matrilineages are descent groups that assign a person specific relatives whose relatedness is traced through the female. Rights to inheritance and land use are assigned to female descendants. A person's clan affiliation is the same as his or her mother's. Women, while enjoying higher status because of their access to resources, have greater autonomy and authority but generally do not hold leadership positions that women's brothers or fathers do. Women are accorded more respect and are more likely to be consulted regarding the welfare of the group.

Brighton Reservation

Because Alice Snow lives at Brighton Reservation, most of her experience relates to Brighton. She collects most of her herbs from around Brighton and gets most of the treatments for the people there. To get a better sense of Alice's world, let us take a closer look at Brighton's history, places, and people.

The Brighton Reservation began in 1938, when the Seminoles living around the northern shore of Lake Okeechobee were given land in Glades County. The Creek-speaking people living in camps in the area moved onto the reservation over the next thirty years. Eventually, they possessed 35,805 acres of pastureland. In the 1940s, a cattle program was inaugurated to help the new residents make the transition from a hunting and gathering society to an agricultural/wage economy. Later, citrus and sugar cane were planted to provide additional tribal income and employment.

Vast pasturelands, equidistant from Okeechobee and Moore Haven, cradle the Brighton community. Two main roads divide the community, while a water tower serves as a landmark at the intersection. Concrete-block houses are arranged in the traditional dispersed settlement style, with only two areas of dense clusters breaking the pattern. Neighbors are often grouped by close kin and clan members. Administrative offices, a gym, rodeo arena, 4-H barn, library, education building, youth center, senior center, police department, nursery, and clinic comprise the main part of the community. Away from the center are the cattle and range administrative building and two Baptist churches. A recreational vehicle park, owned by the Tribe but operated by outsiders, flanks the southern edge. A bingo hall, smoke shop, drive-through convenience store, two cafés, and three craft shops operated by local residents are distributed along the main road of the reservation.

Population

A census taken on August 2, 1995, indicated 506 residents in the community. Of that number, 389 (77 percent) were registered members of the Seminole Tribe of Florida.[8] The other 117 individuals (23 percent) were nontribal members and American Indians holding membership in other tribal organizations or people of European American, African American, or Mexican American heritage. The non-Indian population living on the reservation includes spouses, those cohabiting with Seminoles, and the children of these individuals. Increasing interaction with the general population has led to intermarriage with outsiders, changing the population's character by introducing different cultural attributes.

Economy

Most of the adults (68 percent) interviewed in a random sample taken in 1995 worked for the tribal government or the U.S. government (Bureau of Indian Affairs, or BIA, and other agencies).[9] They consider themselves employees of the Tribe because they are hired through the Tribe and receive checks from that entity. According to the 1990 U.S. census, administrative, support, and service occupations employed 47 percent of those over the age of sixteen. Agricultural jobs ranked next, employing 17 percent of the people. The census is consistent with the survey since the Tribe runs agricultural programs on the reservation. Interview participants generated income in a variety of informal ways. Women (15 percent) sell crafts: beadwork, dolls, and sewing. Men (15 percent) sell products from the cabbage palmetto (*Sabal palmetto* Walt.). The unopened fronds, or buds, are used for Christian Lenten ceremonies, while the fronds are used for the roofs of chickees. The heart of the palm is cooked as "swamp cabbage," and the trees themselves are sold for landscaping. Seven percent of the sample listed building chickees as a way they make money. Ten percent believed that they made money from playing bingo.

Bingo and subsequent gaming activities are profitable for the Tribe. By 1999, most of the government programs were phased out and the tribal government had taken over funding all of the programs except the health clinic, which is provided through treaty agreements. The success of the

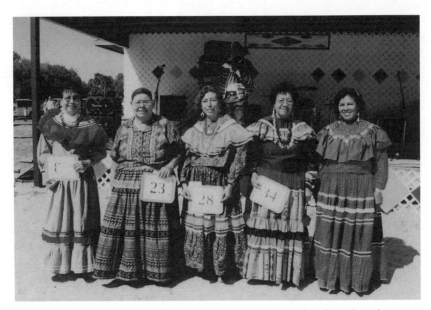

The Seminole Tribe keeps traditional crafts flourishing within the culture by sponsoring dress contests at Brighton Field Days. In this "old-fashioned" dress contest, contestants vie for cash prizes by modeling the dresses they have sewn. Alice frequently designs and creates new dresses for such contests. In this photo from the late 1990s, Mable Haught, Alice, Onnie Osceola, Frances Osceola from the Miccosukee reservation on the Tamiami Trail, and Maggie Henry Garcia from Tampa are the winners. Photograph courtesy of the *Seminole Tribune.*

gaming operations in Tampa, Hollywood, Immokalee, and Brighton brought the Seminoles into self-sufficiency. They are no longer reliant on outside funding to meet their needs. In addition to individual dividends, the tribal government is now able to provide increased infrastructure for the communities. Seniors may request restoration of their aging homes. Community members receive new housing or additions and improvements on their existing homes. Trips to festivals and tournaments reward Tribe members in special circumstances, such as seniors, ball teams, and students. With the help of dividends, working members are now at middle-class income status. They can afford new material goods and pay increased income tax.

Social Structure

Traditional social structure was built around a matrilineal matrilocal system based on clans similar to other southeastern Indian cultures.[10] The basic social unit was an extended family camp of the mother's clan, with the mother's brother, rather than the biological father, serving as disciplinarian to the children. Today, the role of the mother's brother in child rearing is greatly reduced, yet the clan system persists in associations and to some degree in residence patterns. Major clans still in existence are Bird,[11] Panther, Deer, Otter, Snake, Old Town, Bear, and Wind. Clan exogamy dictates that individuals marry someone from a different clan. Traditionally, Bird clan members were the tribal leaders, and the Panther clan was responsible for the medicine bundles and healing. The sacred medicine continues to be the duty of the Panthers, but leadership roles are available to all clans. Ironically, Bird members continue to dominate tribal elections.[12]

Many residents over the age of thirty remember spending their early years living in chickees, the traditional open houses that have been built since the nineteenth century. Today, all reservation residents live in concrete-block houses or mobile homes, though many maintain a chickee in their yards for storage or occasional outdoor living.

Language

Although Creek is the traditional language spoken at Brighton, residents continually express dismay that the younger generation is not speaking it. Forty-six percent of the adults randomly sampled in 1995 still spoke Creek fluently in addition to English.[13] The youngest speaker of Creek was a twenty-seven-year-old female. Some younger persons understand but do not speak the language. Most young parents do not speak Creek in the home.

Religion

The yearly Green Corn Dance (*eshvyvtketv*) maintains ties to traditional religion. The ceremony is central to keeping the medicine bundles and is a symbol of renewal and health for the people. The Green Corn Dance is the celebration of the ripening of the corn and usually occurs in June. A week is set aside to allow participation in fasting and dancing in a remote area. During the event, men are purified through scratching and fasting. Combs, once made of gar teeth but now made of needles, are scraped along the men's arms. The loss of blood from the scratches is symbolic of purification. Women are not scratched because they are purified monthly through menstruation.

The sacred medicine bundles handled by the *heles pocase* of the Panther clan are an integral part of the renewal and healing at the ceremony. It is a time for inspection of the bundles and renewal of their medicinal and protective powers. Traditional Seminole religion incorporates a belief in Hesaketvmesē, or Breathmaker, who instills the power into the medicine bundles. To the existing Green Corn Dance, a ritual of thanksgiving and purification, has been overlaid a belief in Christianity, mostly Baptist. Even people who only attend the Green Corn Dance may at some time in their life affiliate with one of two Indian Baptist churches on the reservation.

The first permanent group of Christian believers was established on the reservation during the 1930s, and attendance peaked by 1945.[14] After the introduction of the Southern Baptist religion, many converts abandoned the traditional Green Corn Dance. The Indian medicine used in the ritual is still important to the many Christians who visit the dance just to receive the medicine for use at home. Other traditional medicine is part of community life, enjoying the support of the medical clinic and behavioral health services.

Education

In 1939, Mr. and Mrs. William D. Boehmer, two white teachers hired by the federal government, established a country day school on the reservation. A bus would visit the scattered camps to bring the children to school. The student population outgrew the school, and it closed in 1954.[15] Students were transferred to local Glades County schools. During these years, before the integration of local county schools, Indian students were assigned to local, mostly black schools. The Seminoles soon realized that the education in those schools was inferior and refused to send their children there. After fighting to attend their county's white schools, the Seminoles came to believe that those schools, too, discriminated against Indian children. As a result, the Tribe contracted to send their children to schools in the adjacent county. This worked well until the home county administrators learned they would receive federal funds for each Indian child and sought to re-enroll them. The Brighton residents would have no part of this switch. When the home county threatened to prohibit Okeechobee County school buses from crossing Glades County lines to pick up Indian students, the Tribe quickly purchased its own school buses to transport the children to the selected schools. These actions and increased schooling indicate how important education is to the Seminoles. Many residents have finished high school, while others have college educations and advanced degrees.

Education, together with intermarriage and Christianity, weakened the clan system and broke down the traditional roles of the matrilineal kinship system. The mother's brother no longer has the position of authority within the family, and, in some cases, the father's authority has not been firmly established.

Social and Physical Concerns

Some concerns involve children who receive low grades, miss a lot of school, or drop out of school. Other concerns involve drug-related activities in school and on the reservation.

The high incidence of alcohol abuse led tribal leaders to apply for a demonstration grant[16] in 1973 and initiate a prevention program (the Seminole Tribe Empowerment Program) in the 1990s. Alcohol abuse and alcohol-related accidents touch the entire community. In response, other prevention programs and recovering alcoholics in the community promote alcohol-free activities. The Tribe has also refurbished a house for the use of the recovering community.

In the health arena, many Seminoles suffer from diabetes mellitus, or type II adult-onset diabetes.[17] From 1994 to 1995, approximately six to eight persons were on dialysis from renal failure attributed to diabetes. In 1998, the clinic on the reservation was seeing eighty diabetic patients (about 20 percent of the Brighton Seminole population).[18]

Despite new interactions with outsiders, the Brighton community is very reluctant to tell others about many aspects of their culture, including the practice of medicine and the training of Indian doctors. Although sensitive to community concerns, the tribal government has supported Alice with funds to develop this book on Seminole traditional medicine.

Alice petitioned the tribal council to fund activities to promote, gather, and teach Indian medicine at the reservations, saying:

I would like to be a full-time employee of the Seminole Tribal Council specializing in managing tribal members' requests for traditional medicine. Throughout my life I have served my community as liaison between Indian doctor and tribal members. I have received requests throughout the day and night; heard individuals describe what is wrong with them; contacted the Indian doctor; gathered the herbs that he needed; prepared the herbs; driven to the doctor's residence; either waited or returned for the medicine to be treated; provided the material; and finally taken the medicine to the member and relayed the directions and restrictions.

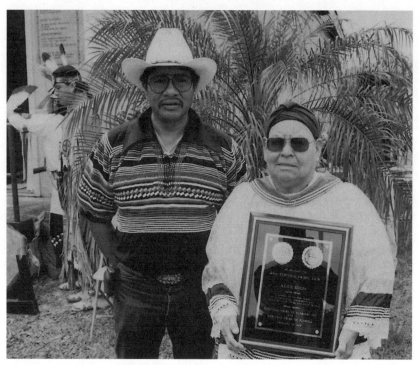

Mitchell Cypress, president of the Seminole Tribe, presents Alice with a plaque denoting that the twenty-eighth Seminole Tribal Fair, in February 1999, was dedicated to her "in appreciation for years of outstanding leadership and guidance of [her] tribe and [her] people." Photograph courtesy of the *Seminole Tribune*.

In the past I have provided these services willingly and freely, using my own time and money for gas. I am proposing that a position be created for me in the community so that I may continue to provide this service to the community. At present, I am employed as a granny for the Head Start program for the Brighton community. As a full-time employee, I cannot respond to the members' requests when they need me, because of working, the time it takes to plan a day off, and the fact that I am trying to reduce my workload. I am an elder and cannot work full-time and meet the requests for medicine. When I hear a member crying that they need medicine, and I cannot leave my job or have to wait until I get time off, I feel badly that I cannot help the person. If I were to concentrate my efforts full-time on the medicine, I could provide the medicine when the person needs it. I am qualified to do this job because I speak Creek and Mikasuki. I know the most herbs used and how to pick and prepare them.

I want the tribal council to sponsor my work with the medicine. The *este-hvtke* who work with the program don't allow Seminole workers to do the medicine the way we did in the past. Also, it takes too long to help the people.

In addition to gathering and getting the medicine treated, I would be willing to teach others about the herbs for that day when I am gone. I would also like to arrange meetings between doctors and tribal members who want to learn the songs. If the members were sincere about learning then I would plan the meeting time and place and provide herbs for the members to learn to identify.

In summary, I would like the tribe to support my efforts to continue to provide Indian medicine to the people and to begin training younger members in the medicine. With the support, I can continue to meet my expenses and provide a service to members unable to drive or buy hogs and material.

Alice was granted the request.

Brighton residents consider themselves progressive, appreciating education, new technologies, and improved relationships with the dominant culture. The Seminole Tribe of Florida is no longer composed of quaint people clinging to a passing lifestyle, but of survivors of a cultural upheaval that has blended the complex structures of an earlier life with the contemporary. Their recent acculturation and self-determination place them on the cusp of yet another stage of culture change—the economic and educational trappings of middle-class America.

2

Seminole Traditional Medicine

♦♦♦♦♦♦♦♦♦♦♦♦♦♦♦♦♦♦♦

Alice Snow's knowledge of Indian medicine comes from her experience identifying plants and their properties. The medicinal plants used by native healers reflect a long-term, systematic, tested observation of nature. Indian medicine falls under the category of ethnomedicine, which describes how indigenous people practice healing and what methods they use. Ethnobotanist Gary J. Martin elaborates on the definition, saying, "*Ethno* is a popular prefix these days, because it is a short way of saying 'that's the way other people look at the world.'"[1] When biomedical scientists study the healing practices of other cultures, they gain valuable clues to plant properties already tested through multiple generations of use.[2] Preserving indigenous knowledge becomes even more important.

Despite the loss of many elements of traditional life, native medicine is still practiced among the Seminoles. From 1950 to 1952, William Sturtevant interviewed and recorded the ethnomedicine of Josie Billie, a Miccosukee Indian doctor and medicine man. There have been changes in the medicine since that study, but Seminole medicine is still in use throughout the reservation system. In the summer of 1998, for instance, medicine man and Indian doctor Bobby Henry performed a rain ceremony to quench the rain-starved southeastern United States and extinguish the wildfires that plagued Florida.[3] Other examples abound: Relatives visit a tribal elder who is a patient at the local hospital, bringing a freshly brewed concoction of herbal medicine, which she surreptitiously hides under her bed. When a friend experiences dizziness, Alice consults a local Indian doctor regarding preparations for comfort and cure. Babies wear tiny sacks of white material or suede, pinned to their shirt or on a necklace of white beads to protect them in their first years of life. The Behavior Health Program, which deals with alcohol abuse in the community, has stacks of cloth bolts on a file cabinet awaiting measurement to reward an Indian doctor for his services in making "on the wagon" medicine.

Indian medicine comprises a minimum of five elements: the patient (*este-enokkv*), the doctors and collectors (*heles-hayvlke*), the herbs (*rvkvpv*), the diagnosis, and the treatment or songs. The person who is ill may request help, or a relative, usually a mother or sister, may request a treatment. He or she may call the doctor directly or consult a collector, who will contact the doctor. The doctor agrees to treat, or "fix," the medicine, and describe the process that varies according to what is wrong with the patient. Questions about dreams or other events surrounding the ill person may be asked.

The following account, taken from my field notes, describes Alice's visit to an Indian doctor for the continued healing of her knee following surgery.

Alice took bay (*tolv*), ice plant (*hetotvpe*), ginseng (*heles-hvtke*), and willow (*akwanv*) to a doctor. The doctor's daughter acted as an intermediary, asking Alice what she wanted. She was getting two medicines: one to heal her knee following replacement surgery and the other for a sharp pain that she sometimes felt in her leg when she moved it. Speaking in Mikasuki, she said she had one operation and the knee got infected again. She was reoperated on and had to go to a nursing home for five weeks. The knee didn't heal well. Another Indian doctor treated her once after surgery on her other knee, and it didn't work. The other doctor had treated the knee with hot medicine. After speaking to her father, the daughter said it would not heal fast enough unless he treated it with cool medicine.

He prepared the medicine in the back room while we waited and visited with the daughter in the living room. Although we could not see or hear him, the Indian doctor sang the songs and blew in the medicine, which gave the treatment its healing properties. After about an hour, the daughter brought Alice the medicine with the instructions from the Indian doctor. She was told to follow this prescription: During the first four days of using the cool medicine, she was to have no hot stuff, like coffee, unless it was lukewarm. She must not leave the coolness of the house and go in the hot sun. She could drive or ride in a car the day after taking the medicine. She had to stay inside until then.

For the pain, she was not to eat meat from four-legged animals if the bones were cooked with it. If the meat was removed from the bone before cooking, she could have beef or pork. She could eat chicken and fish. Alice said, "It is hard to go out to eat when a person is on Indian medicine."

Finally, the daughter told Alice what the doctor required in return for fixing the medicine. Alice gave her four yards of yellow material for the knee treatment and four yards of red material for the pain medicine.

Alice asked about another treatment. She had dreamed that someone died. So that the dream wouldn't come true, she asked for some more medicine to be treated. It was a bundle of bay branches and leaves (*tolv*). She was told to burn the bundle and let the smoke waft over her. She was not to watch television for one day. Since this treatment was an afterthought, she had not brought any black material to give the doctor. We went out to the local shops to find the material. Not finding any, she looked for a black towel or T-shirt. We found only a black T-shirt with a Chicago White Sox emblem on it, so she purchased it. She got an XL, which she thought would be the right size for the doctor. When she took the shirt back to him, he looked it over and said okay. Because it wasn't yardage, he had to approve it, but he liked the design. He took the shirt and the bay leaves to the back room to sing the songs. It took him about forty minutes to treat the leaves for bad dreams.

Another example of a treatment is one to stop drinking alcohol. When a son, daughter, or sibling has been drinking too much, a mother or sister will most likely request *vwotickv*, or "on the wagon" medicine for that person. When the mother requests the medicine and instructs the offspring to take it, the drinker is compelled to take the medicine out of tradition. In the case of "on the wagon" medicine, the doctor wants to know who will take the medicine. If the doctor thinks that there is little chance that the patient will comply with the restrictions that go along with the medicine, he or she is likely to refuse to fix the medicine. The prevailing belief is that breaking the restrictions while using the medicine causes harm to come to the doctor, as well as causing a severe relapse for the patient. Not everyone is a good candidate for treatment.

If the doctor deems the patient suitable, he or she instructs the intermediary to collect specific medicines, usually in a specific order. The medicines are collected fresh from the local woods, broken up into smaller pieces, and the herbs are taken—either in water or dry—to the doctor to be "fixed."

Doctors use many songs to instill power in the medicine. The songs are lengthy and most sung in the Creek/Muskogee language. Apprenticeship and repetitious singing with traditional healers are the only way to maintain this cultural tradition, for the songs are guarded as secret from the outside world and important in ceremony.[4] A Seminole interested in becoming a doctor must study long and memorize the songs aurally. Audiotaping of the singing is prohibited, even when teaching someone to become a doctor. The songs do not change, but treatments can vary as to the type and number of herbs, of goods exchanged for services, and of restrictions for the patient.

Sturtevant distinguishes between the Indian doctor and the medicine man. Both are high-prestige, respected positions, with the Indian doctor earning his position from long practice and efficacy of treatments. The medicine man is responsible for the keeping of the sacred medicine bundles used at the Green Corn Dance. Frequently the roles are combined in one man, but only a man from the Panther clan may be the keeper of the medicine bundles.

Much of the healing instruction is secret. Josie Billie, a healer of the past, reported spending four years in observation, fasting, and studying to become a doctor. He gained his reputation as an effective healer only after a long practice, the respect that comes with age, and the death of other healers.[5]

Josie Billie described his intensive training to become an Indian doctor at the beginning of the century. He said that the doctor must begin at an early age before he is married. It takes many years of experience before a doctor is recognized and has a busy practice. In those times, doctoring school was called *boosketau* (Creek: *posketv*), which means "to fast."[6] Training involved fasting, sweating, using emetics for purification, and learning through dreams, which are considered omens. The main focus of the formal "doctor" school is to learn the long and difficult songs, the diagnoses, and the various treatments. Students are expected to learn about the medicinal herbs outside the school. Josie Billie stated that the songs are more important than the plants. He believed that water treated by the songs could be a curative, even without the plants.[7]

After the doctor agrees to treat the patient, he or she requests specific herbs (*heleswv*),[8] as well as the gift expected in exchange for services rendered (such as a piece of cloth or sometimes a chicken, hog, ax, knife, or gun). Because their training is free, the doctors are expected to perform their service for free, accepting gifts rather than payments. Although some doctors do accept money at times, Alice believes that accepting money will render the treatment ineffective. She is critical of those who prepare medicine to make a monetary profit. When the diagnosis is complete, the collector gathers the herbs and the gift.

Tribal officials view Seminole medicine as an important part of their culture and support it through programs and funding. Elderly Indian doctors continue to provide instruction for interested Seminoles. Traditionally, the doctors do not recruit students, but rather students must come to them and ask to learn the medicine. It is unknown whether the training is still as rigorous as in the past.

Today, Seminole traditional medicine coexists with biomedicine in the communities of the Seminole Tribe of Florida. Traditional medicine augments and complements procedures and treatments used. In clinical programs, health care workers are encouraged to understand and to promote the use of traditional medicine, in addition to the healing regimen of the biomedical doctors and nurses. In 1999 Brighton Seminole elders spoke to health care workers at a local hospital to help them understand Seminole practices. Commenting on this discussion, Alice said, "I told them, 'Sometimes our people don't eat the hospital food and you get worried. But you don't know we are also on Indian medicine that restricts us from eating some foods.' They agreed to do whatever they could for those patients to help them out."

Common Health Problems

In 1944, Robert Greenlee wrote that the following illnesses were the most frequently reported by the people at the time: digestive disorders, arthritis, poor teeth, influenza and colds, malaria, diarrhea, hookworm, venereal disease, and alcohol use. Later Sturtevant found reports of the relatively good health of the Seminole and summarized some of the most prevalent health conditions from government reports.[9] He listed "infant mortality, colds, hookworm, tooth decay, pneumonia, influenza, dysentery, chicken pox, measles, whooping cough, and mumps." Four cases of diabetes were listed, foreshadowing the major health concern that plagues the tribe into the new century. Except for treatments for arthritis and alcohol abuse, Seminole traditional medicine in the past and Alice's list of treatments address associated symptoms of these diseases, not the diseases themselves. The disease categories in this section refer to the biomedical names for health problems, not to the Seminole view of ailments, which is discussed later.

Causes of Disease

Informal tribal publications list five causes of disease: soul loss, when the soul fails to return to the body after dreaming; agents in the form of spirits of animals, such as a monkey, and natural forces, like lightning; sorcery, when a Seminole casts an evil spell on another person; the intrusion of a foreign object in the body; and wounds from cuts, gunshots, or bites. Over the years, fewer and fewer illnesses have been attributed to these causes. Soul loss, sorcery, and intrusion are seldom referred to in the community.

Alice's Categories of Treatment

Back in the 1940s, Greenlee organized treatments as follows: those that cured bodily ills, those that helped maintain health and relationships, those preventing soul loss, and mysterious mental ailments. Medicine to maintain health included death medicine, tobacco to ward off danger from other people, and love potions. He mentioned that black magic, or harmful medicine, was no longer used.

To come up with the categories of treatment that Alice uses today, she and I sat down with all the written treatments before us. After we discussed the first one, I asked about the second, "Is this treatment like the first one, or is it different?" We did this for all the treatments until we had several separate piles. We then arranged the piles in groups that were alike in some way. Finally, we had a classification of the different treatments, a taxonomy. (For details, see the accompanying table.)

The three main categories were those concerning the annual Green Corn Dance, which is the domain of male medicine men (*heles pocase*), treatments regarding prevention, and treatments regarding healing, both of which are the domain of the doctor (*heles hayv*). This book is concerned only with the treatments prescribed by the *heles hayv*. A *heles pocase* usually is also a *heles hayv*, but few doctors become the keepers of the medicine bundles. No woman may keep the medicine bundles, but many have become Indian doctors.

Alice's list of treatments reflects current Seminole views about the causes of sickness, which differ greatly from the older tradition described in the previous section. According to Sturtevant, that tradition, with its many natural and supernatural causal agents, was hard to systematize, presenting "such difficulties that the conclusion is inescapable that even the doctors themselves have only vague and often inconsistent ideas about the manner in which these causes operate."[10]

Most of the treatments cited by Josie Billie in the 1950s related to such disease agents as living animals or their ghosts, natural phenomena, such as fire and the supernatural, and some social causes. Few of these treatments persist today, perhaps reflecting the inclusion of biomedical treatment into the Seminole healing system. Whereas Sturtevant recorded forty-six treatments (52 percent) for illnesses said to be caused by events or animals, Alice knew only one full treatment—for monkey sickness—although she had heard of several sicknesses related to animals and the supernatural.[11] She said, "Whatever kind of animal you dream of is the kind that is causing the sickness. If you dream about black animals, like the bear, you see them and are not able to get away from them in your dream. From the size and the number you can tell how it makes you sick." Today, the illness called alligator sickness is not related to a dream but rather to an alligator bite.

Alice was familiar with some of the information on the little people (*este-lopocke*),[12] a supernatural causal agent, but had not had personal experience with treatment for the condition. She did report seeing the little people around her bed once when she was hospitalized with a severe illness. She says simply that they are all around but appear infrequently, most likely when someone is sick. They live in bundles of needles on the branches of pine trees. The bundles or bark from the tree, considered very powerful, are used in curing mental illnesses.

I asked Alice to show me where the little people live, because I was not familiar with the phenomenon. After a few months, she reported finding one, and she took me to see it about sixty miles from her home, just south of Holopaw, Florida. Very clearly, a gnarl had formed on a branch, as pictured in color photo 6. Although she said it was important to get the needle bundle, I remarked that taking the bundle would eliminate a very scarce resource and that being very high in the tree it would be hard to get. It was then that she told me that if it were unreachable, the bark would suffice.

Alice uses several treatments that are related to social issues, such as medicine to protect a baby from its father's touch (in the case of his adultery), but this comprises only 5 percent of her repertoire. Many of her treatments deal with specific symptoms, and only two—stroke medicine and hysterectomy—relate to Western diagnoses. Stroke medicine is sought as an adjunct to the Western treatment when the latter does not appear to help the patient; it is also used to hasten healing. Alice does not usually use the Western diagnosis; she just describes the symptoms to the Indian doctor, as when she seeks treatment for a patient's speeding heart. This signals a shift from the past and an integration of the medicine into modern therapy.

One category of treatment is related to sleep and bad dreams. Alice said such treatments are to be taken "if you like to sleep all the time and for bad dreams." They differ as to the herbs to be taken and songs to be sung. They are alike in relating to the problem of sleep and dreams. As Alice explained, the Indian doctors base the treatments upon the patient's dreams and sleep experiences:

> The treatment and songs are determined by the questions that the medicine doctor asks you. He will ask you what kind of dream you had or what kind of animals are in the dream. He also wants to know the person you dreamed about. Then he will know what treatment to use.[13]

> Indian doctors ask you that all the time when you are sick. They ask, "What kind of dream did she have?" My niece said she had a pain right across the stomach that was kind of hard. The doctor asked, "Is the stomach making some kind of growling?" I said I didn't know, and he didn't tell me what medicine to get. I said I would get back with him, but I never did, because my niece changed her mind.

Alice continued, giving examples of two of her own dreams:

> I am going to use my grandmother and mother when they died. When I dreamed about them I see them cooking a lot of food. When they finish cooking and they start to eat, they ask you to eat with them. You are kind of hungry, too, and you would like to eat. They are trying to take your spirit. And you even might die later. If you eat with them, then you have to take the medicine. If you don't and you wake up, you don't need the medicine.

> I had a lot of dreams when my husband died. I would see him and he was *hace* [drunk], not real *hace*, but he was drinking all the time. He was driving a big old truck. He asked me to go drinking with him. But I said no. Even if I did drive with him, I didn't drink. I woke up each time, before I started drinking [in the dream]. Maybe the Lord

was saying, "Hey, you don't do that." I didn't take the medicine after that because I didn't go drinking with him. If I had started drinking with him in the dream, I would have taken the medicine.

Dreams are thus used two ways: animals in a dream are diagnostics, and dream situations can be harbingers of danger.[14] Either way, they require treatment with medicine to effect a cure or return to a state of equilibrium.

Another category of Seminole medicine includes treatments to prevent illness or for protection as well as those that are used to heal sickness. An overlapping category seems to be one that creates balance or aids in heal-

Table 1. Classification of treatments in Alice's repertoire

Ceremonial medicine bundles
    Continued well-being
    Protection during warfare
    Curing from war-related injury

Prevention		
Health	Treatments for babies	
	Treatment for women	
	Treatment for pregnant women	
Protection after event	Protect baby from father's touch	
	Death medicine	
Dream	Treatment for bad dreams	
	Treatment for worry	
Sleep-related	Treatment for not being able to sleep	
	Treatment for sleeping too much	
Operation-related	Cool medicine	
	Treatment for hysterectomy	

Healing		
Animal-caused sickness	Treatment for alligator bite	
Animal-behavior sickness	Treatment for monkey sickness	
Sickness/ailment cure	"On the wagon" medicine	
	Pain treatments	
	Ear treatment	
	Treatment for baby who cries all the time	
	Treatment for baby who won't eat	
	Treatment for blackout or shortness of breath	
	Treatment for a speeding heart	
	Treatment for stroke	

ing secondary conditions. These categories tend to involve hot and cold principles. For example, cold medicine is used to prevent problems following an operation. Because the tools used in the operation are heated in the sterilization process, the cold medicine provides a protective balance. Alice described how Indian medicine supplements Western medicine in such circumstances: "I used Indian medicine after I had a gall bladder operation. I used pain pills after the surgery and it helped for a few hours, but after a while it comes back. Indian medicine makes it go."

Animal-related treatments tend to be named for the cause of the sickness, which mainly appears in dreams, or the person has a peculiar behavior that is like the animal's. Alice explained that monkey sickness is the mimicking of a monkey's grooming behavior: the individual picks at the skin or hair, then moves the hand to the nose and mouth. Sturtevant employs a similar definition for this condition but adds that the eyes are enlarged and the babies and adults are feverish. Fever and enlarged eyes were not a part of Alice's description. While Josie Billie treated monkey sickness by using sassafras that had been heated, Alice's treatments did not.

The effectiveness of traditional, or ethnomedical, treatments has often been attributed to the placebo effect. The belief in a medicine's efficacy and the symbols of healing such as the white lab coat or herb punch set up conditions for psychological healing, which enhances the physiological cure. Daniel Moerman, who has studied the placebo effect of surgery for heart patients, states that "neither native therapists nor their patients saw pharmaceuticals as any more important in therapy than the song, dance, and din that accompanied treatment."[15] Although Seminole medicine is believed to get its power from the infusion of the supernatural through chants, that does not negate the importance of active properties in the herbs themselves. To examine the pharmaceutical use of Seminole herbs, we now turn to ethnobotany, or native plant use.

3

The Traditional Use of Plants

◆◆◆◆◆◆◆◆◆◆◆◆◆◆◆◆◆◆◆

Traditional uses of plants have worldwide interest to those who study health problems today. Ethnobotanists learn how people classify and identify plants, what properties each plant has, and the relationship between people and plants. Local or indigenous people have accumulated their healing information through empirical observation and from enculturation from parents and peers. Ethnobotany represents a growing academic field as we search for cures for modern diseases. Yet as more and more traditional healers die and folk remedies disappear into the biomedical tradition, knowledge of the relationship between the animal and plant world is disappearing.

The loss of biodiversity throughout the world and the extinction of species are limiting factors in botanical research. Nevertheless, the potential is enormous, for only 10 percent of the world's quarter million flowering species of plants have been tested for their medicinal properties.[1] In 1973 the chemical compounds from higher plant species made up about a quarter of prescription drugs sold in the United States.[2] Out of 199 medicinal plants such as quinine, digitoxin, and reserpine, 153 were found because they were used in indigenous healing practices.[3] Use of plant compounds in prescription drugs is big business, valued in 1980 in the United States at approximately $8 billion.[4] Drug companies continue to explore the active properties of plants worldwide. By examining preparations that indigenous people have tested for years, scientists hope to find new drugs for treatment of diseases such as cancer and AIDS.

One effective herb that has been used by the Seminoles is *welanv* (*Chenopodium ambrosiodes*). Roots mixed in water are used as an astringent after a person stops using an Indian treatment lasting four months, such as *vwotickv*. Alice watched this herb being prepared and used: The roots are selected and put in water, and the doctor fixes the mixture with a song. The person drinks a little bit four times, then washes his or her face, arms, and legs. Josie Billie used this treatment for worm sickness. Children between the ages of ten and twelve are most likely to have the condition, caused by crawling on the ground and eating some dirt or raw food. The afflicted child looks pale and tired but has a large appetite—symptoms consistent with intestinal worms. Josie Billie used the herb by boiling the plant in water, treating the mixture with the proper chant, and having the patient drink it. In 1947, the herb was reported to be an effective anthelmintic, or worm remedy.[5] Because of advances in Western medicine and the fact that most children wear shoes nowadays, intestinal worms are less of a problem, reducing the need for this treatment.

Alice knows the identity of some of the old medicines, such as *wotko elupe* (literally "raccoon liver"; botanical name, *Stenandrium floridanum*). However, she does not remember how *wotko elupe* was used. Josie Billie reported it as one ingredient in a charm to stop a baby from crying. (The charm was a small bag of white cloth filled with a variety of herbs such as *heles-hvtke* [ginseng], *tolv* [bay], and *vcenv* [cedar].) The cause of the crying was said to be bad dreams usually involving a raccoon or opossum. *Wotko elupe* was probably used because of its relationship to the animal in the dream.

Recently, herbal remedies have made a modest comeback among the general population. For example, St. John's Wort (*Hypericum perforatum*) is a natural remedy for depression that some people use as a substitute for the frequently prescribed Prozac. A related species, *Hypericum aspalathoides,* is found in the pinelands and prairies of Florida. Although Alice has not used it in treatments and cannot remember its Creek name, she saw an Indian doctor collect it once and can now recognize it. She describes this herb as *envrke nokke heleswv* (stomach pain medicine).

Several well-known herbs she uses appear among Western pharmaceuticals. *Akwanv* (Carolina willow, or *Salix amphibia*) is utilized in many Seminole treatments. The bark is known to contain salicylates, a precursor of the ingredient acetasalicylic acid in aspirin.[6] Alice recognizes the elderberry or *coskelpv* (*Sambucus simpsonii* Rehder), which grows in abundance around swampy areas, as a medicine used in the past. She has not been called upon to collect it, yet laboratory tests at Hadasah-Hebrew University Medical Center at Ein Karem, Israel, suggest it may have possibilities as a curative for flu. Elderberries have frequently been used as a folk remedy for coughs, colds, fevers, and runny noses. Syrup and lozenges that contain the compounds in elderberries are being marketed as Sambucol.[7]

One herb used frequently in Seminole medicine is *heles-hvtke*, translated as "white medicine" (ginseng, or *Panax quinquefolium*). This herb is used by many cultures as part of their health regimen. The dried root, which is white when peeled, is dissolved in water to relieve pain on mucous membranes, to improve digestion, or to act as an aphrodisiac. It is believed to aid in the cure of appendicitis, body weakness, headache, lumbago, rheumatism, and sciatica. Because it is an antispasmodic, ginseng may be useful for whooping cough, asthma, gastroenteric indigestion, and a weak heart. It has been listed both as a stimulant and as a mild sedative. As early as 1657, Father Jartoux reported American Indians in the Ozarks and Blue Ridge Mountains using ginseng as medicine.[8]

Some parts of the plants used by Alice, such as the berries of mistletoe and the roots of the water hemlock, are poisonous. Poisons may be useful to the plant's survival in warding off herbivores and pests, but when administered in minute doses, they can be more therapeutic than toxic.[9] Herbalists suggest that the use of mistletoe stems and leaves slows the heart rate and dilates the arteries to lower blood pressure; this is consistent with Seminole doctors' use of small amounts of mistletoe in the supplementary treatment for stroke patients. Since Seminole treatments are often used as body washes on the skin, the dosage may be absorbed though the skin like nicotine and nitroglycerine patches used in biomedical pharmaceutics.

Another body wash or transdermal application is the arthritis treatment using the poisonous, tuberlike roots of the water hemlock (*Cicuta maculata*). When used in Seminole medicine, these roots are applied as an astringent to the skin but are not consumed. In Alice's description of cool medicine (p. 67), *akwanv* or willow bark is used as a wash to treat the area of an incision following surgery. Daniel Moerman states that natural salicylates in willow bark are more toxic than the chemical in aspirin, but the natural chemical is easily absorbed through the skin.[10] In fact, natural salicylates are used in sports creams to relieve pain from muscle aches. This suggests that Seminole medicine is dependent on active ingredients in the herbs as well as the ritual treatment. The use of body washes has been generally overlooked in the search for cures based on indigenous medicinal practices. Anthropologists Michelle Alexander and Anthony Parades suggest that this application may be more useful in the future in our understanding of the efficacy of traditional medicine, particularly with the increase in the use of patches rather than ingestion in biomedical practices.[11] Indeed, with so many Seminole mixtures being applied as "baths," the greatest healing properties may be in skin absorption.

The mixtures that the Seminole Indians use appear to be sufficiently diluted in proportion and in application to reduce toxic effects. Nevertheless, as noted earlier, Alice believes that Indian medicine may be "too strong" for white people. She described how to use stroke medicine, which contains mistletoe and willow bark: "Use a lot for *este-cate* [literally 'red person' but refers to Indians], but for white persons, just use a little bit, because it will be too strong for them." She judges the strength of the mixture by the depth of the red color that comes from the willow bark in the water. This phenomenon needs to be investigated further; both the mixtures themselves and their potentiating effects need to be analyzed.

Paul Alan Cox, botany professor and dean at Brigham Young University, seeks out traditional healers to find plants beneficial for Western medicine.[12] He likens the use of rituals of flicking ashes before providing the curative or the "spiritual transmission" in Western Samoa to the belief transmitted by doctors wearing white coats in our society. White coats are a symbol of healing that confers comfort and expertise. In the same manner, the infusion of the power of healing into the treatments used by the Seminole represents a similar spiritual transmission.

Diminished Supplies of Herbs

According to Alice, the following plants are hard to find today: *welanv, yamēlikv, passv, svpeyv-lopockuce, svpeyv rakko, cetto heleswv, 'coheceko,* and *aktvpēhv.* Plants were lost when land was cleared on and off the reservation. Fencing now restricts access to some herbs. Because of overharvesting of some of the more popular species, such as ginseng (*Panax quinquefolium*), the natural supply was reported nearly depleted in many of Florida's northern woods by 1953.[13]

Much of the natural ginseng in North America, the oldest being the most desired for its potency, was shipped to China to fill the demands there. It is a slow-growing herb, taking as long as five to seven years for the root to grow large enough to be of use. The age of the plants is determined by counting the number of rings, with the oldest being the most sought after and requiring the lowest dosage.[14] Of course when roots of the plant are needed for medicine, such as *heles-hvtke* and *passv*, the chances of plant reproduction are diminished.

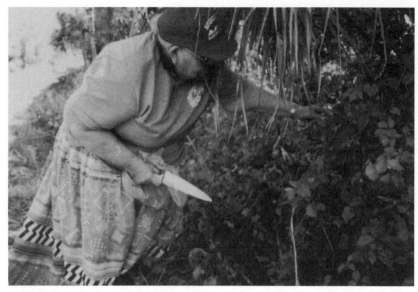

A sharp knife and a bag to hold the medicine make up Alice's plant-gathering tool kit. Photograph by Michael O. James, used courtesy of the photographer.

Some herbs cannot be found during all seasons because they are annuals or they die back following frosts. Alice had to plan gathering some material according to growing seasons or after plants recovered. It is important for herbs to be collected fresh, so she never kept herbs on hand for the scarce season but relied more on searching out the seedling, long before the plant was established, or simply omitted the herb from the mix.

Herbs that are in danger of extinction or that are inconvenient to collect are not cultivated or grown domestically by keepers of the medicine tradition because they believe that all the steps to creating the medicine must remain true to the time-tested gathering methods. When elders at Brighton were approached to begin a medicinal plant garden, they declined, stating that the effectiveness is dependent on gathering in the wild. Hence tradition takes precedence over preservation.

Collection and Preparation of Herbs

Generally the herbs are collected in a specific order. When the treatment includes *tolv*, or red bay, that is collected first. Although there is an effort to collect the herbs in order, it is often impossible because of the diverse locations of the ingredients (*heleswv vtelokv*).[15] Not only must the collector know the herbs, where to find them, and the order of collection, but she or he must know what parts to collect, how much to collect, and any special orientation involved in selecting the specimens (*tolv,* for example, is generally collected from the east side of the tree).

The parts of plants that Alice collects are bark, leaves, stems, and roots—but no flowers or fruit. She identifies each plant based upon her knowledge of the season, the topography, and the plant's overall appearance. She does not need the flower for identification, but wild flower books and botanical taxonomies rely more heavily on the flower than the parts she considers important. When Alice and I could not pin down the botanical name of a plant, we traveled to the herbarium at the University of Florida. Sometimes, when shown the blossom preserved with the plant at the herbarium, she would say, "Oh, yes. That's what it looks like."

Some parts of plants that are collected symbolize the body parts involved in the sickness. In anthropological terms, this is called imitative magic—that is, like treats like. For women's treatments, Alice collects the forks of tree branches from the Carolina ash, ficus, and pine tree, which resemble the legs of a woman. The cure is associated with reproductive organs. The Chippewa are known to search for a divided root in a plant because it resembled the legs of a man.[16]

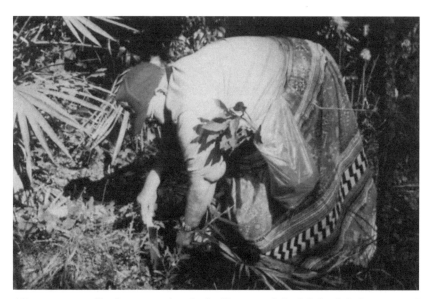

Alice stoops to dig the roots of an herb. Photograph by Michael O. James, used courtesy of the photographer.

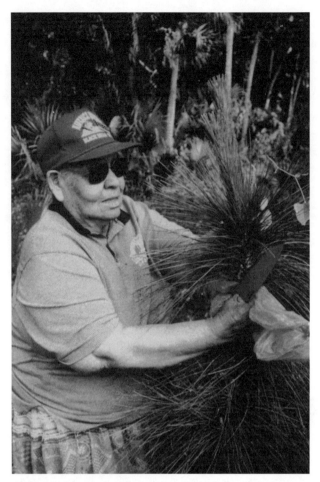

Alice cuts the tip of a pine sapling (*cule*) for a medical treatment. Photograph by Michael O. James, used courtesy of
the photographer.

After the herbs are collected, they must be prepared for use. Some examples of herb preparation have already been provided earlier in the text.
Here is how Alice prepared the herbs for stroke medicine:

Rinse off the roots. Cut the bark of the willow small enough to put it
in the plastic jug opening [one-gallon plastic milk jug]. Put the herbs
in water the same day as collected to make the treatment strong.
Break them all up to get everything into the jug. Fill the jug half full
with water. It is not filled to the top so there will be room to blow air

into the mixture while it's being treated. The doctor uses a reed or straw to blow in the air. If a plant or piece of it is dropped in gathering or preparation, do not pick it up and use it. It is a bad thing to do.

Commonly Used Plants

Among the 205 herbs listed in one source of medicinal plants of Native Americans,[17] Alice recognized 15 (7 percent) as used by the Seminoles. The best known of the Seminole herbs used worldwide include wax myrtle, huckleberry, blue flag or iris, elderberry, button snakeroot, ginseng, gold-

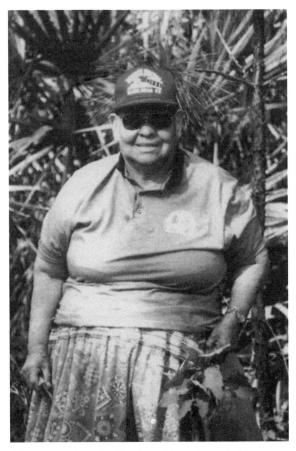

After a morning of collecting, Alice returns to her car with herbs. Photograph by Michael O. James, used courtesy of the photographer.

enrod, mallow, maple, penny royal sage, sassafras, saw palmetto, sumac, sundew, and willow.

William Sturtevant and Robert Greenlee have written the most material about the medicine of the Seminole. Both worked with Mikasuki-speaking medicine men to describe treatments and herbs. Identification of some of the herbs for this book was possible by referring to Sturtevant's earlier work, but many of the herbs he describes may have been lost or Alice was unfamiliar with them. Sturtevant lists about 225 medicinal herbs known by Josie Billie; Alice has 74 herbs in her repertoire (see Appendix A). In a separate study, eight elderly herb collectors at Brighton Reservation recited all the plants they could think of that are used in the medicine.[18] Collectively, these eight women, including Alice, remembered approximately 200 different herbs; the most frequently mentioned were *tolv* and *passv* (button snakeroot, or *Eryngium yucciafolium* Michx.), which were cited by all.

The frequency with which herbs are mentioned relates to their cultural saliency or importance. *Tolv* is universally recognized and is most frequently used in treatments. *Passv* is utilized in few treatments, occurs somewhat rarely, yet may be remembered because of its use in the ceremonial medicine bundles. Earlier reports suggest that the Seminoles used the roots of *passv* as a ceremonial "black drink" or purgative taken before important council deliberations.[19] This would account for its relative scarcity. However, Alice is not familiar with the use of *passv* in "black drink." According to Charles Hudson, *Ilex vomitoria* was used as a purifier in early southeastern Indian ceremonial complexes.[20] But Alice has no knowledge of this use either.

Analyzing the herbs most frequently used by Josie Billie, Sturtevant found that *tolv* was employed in about 31 percent of the cases; *vcenv* (cedar) and *wēso* (sassafras) were both used in about 13 percent; and *akwanv* (willow), *heles-hvtke* (ginseng), *ue-heleswv* (lizard's tail plant), *passv,* and *sakcometo* (button bush) were used between 6 and 10 percent of the time. Among the herbs utilized in the treatments Alice recorded for this book, *tolv* was the most frequently used (70 percent of the time). Next were *akwanv* (37 percent), *ue-heleswv* (26 percent), *heles-hvtke, heles-here* (downy milk pea) (19 percent), *hefepe-nērkv* (bottle gourd seeds) (15 percent), and *lucv-huehkv enhompetv* (gopher apple) (11 percent); the rest were used less than once (4 percent) or twice (7 percent).

Some families of plants range from South Florida to northern climes. Like the Chippewa Indians of Minnesota, Wisconsin, and Canada, the

Seminoles use plants from the goldenrod (*Solidago*) and poplar (*Populus*) families.[21] The Chippewa use goldenrod as an astringent and styptic. The herb contains a volatile oil. Various *Populus* species are used as an aromatic, expectorant, or tonic. The Seminoles trade *tartahkv* (white ash or cottonwood), which is in the *Populus* genus,[22] from more northern areas.

Using techniques from historical linguistics, we can tell something about the longevity of some of the treatments as well as hypothesize about the Seminoles' former environment. Two herbs, *heles-hvtke* (ginseng) and *wēso* (sassafras), do not grow in South Florida, but they are still a part of the Seminole medicine repertoire because of their perceived effectiveness. Both occur naturally in the former territory of the Seminoles—Georgia, Alabama, and North Florida. Now that they live primarily in South Florida, the Seminoles have to import the herbs, usually from Oklahoma.

Native plant use has contributed to Western knowledge of healing, the most notable contribution of the American Indian being quinine still used to treat malaria. Generations have tested herbal remedies and have continued to use them. Therefore, indigenous collectors and doctors have a wealth of knowledge that may be lost without proper respect for them and their teachings.

4

Alice's Story

"When I Was Coming Up . . ."

♦♦♦♦♦♦♦♦♦♦♦♦♦♦♦♦♦♦♦

Alice says she was born September 15, 1922, although that date cannot be confirmed because records were not kept in those days. Years later, when her parents wanted her to qualify for a driver's license, they offered that date so she would be old enough to be tested. She estimates that she was about thirteen at the time, while the legal driving age was fifteen.

Alice was born in an open place in the woods, on land that now makes up Brighton Reservation in Glades County. It was not until 1938 that the land would be set aside for the Seminoles remaining in Florida following the U.S. government's removal of most of the Seminoles to Oklahoma. Sixty years had passed since the Third, and final, Seminole War, which left between 150 and 200 Creek- and Mikasuki-speaking people who had become known as "Seminoles."

Alice was the fifth child of Emma Maudy and Charlie Micco. As an infant she was given the Seminole name *Tefolothokv*, which means "go around each other" or "one passes by." She, like her mother and her mother's mother, would be a member of the Bird clan (*Fuswvlke*). Her older siblings were Charlie Micco, Goby Micco Tiger, Leona Micco Smith, and Cody Micco. She has two younger brothers, Jack and Howard, who are Baptist ministers. Alice tells about her own childhood in the Red Barn area on Brighton Reservation: "Where I grew up was nothing fancy—living in a chickee, sleeping on the platform. And when we were driving, we were riding in the back of the wagon. We didn't go out in the wagon all the time. Most of the time they [her parents] just left us home when they went to town. They didn't have much room in the wagon, I guess. That's why most of the time we stayed home and played around. I guess that is the

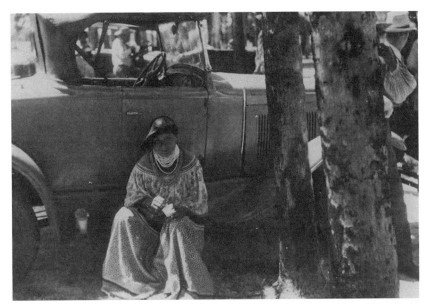

Alice eats ice cream while sitting on the running board of the car her sister Cody won around 1934 or 1935. Photograph from the William D. Boehmer Collection, courtesy of the Department of Anthropology and Genealogy, Seminole Tribe of Florida.

reason our family is close now. We were always in the camp together. Since we left the Red Barn camp we spread out." Alice remembers her childhood as one of play. "We would play any kind of sticks. Like palmetto sticks. Like little horses. We would just have to make a point and play with our hands and cow bones, and back then we didn't have any kind of play stuff. Like the ones they've got today. That's why we had to make our own."

One of the games she played with her brothers and sisters was cow bones (*wakv-torkopohlikv*). A bone from the knee of the cow was used to throw into the soft sand. Different scores were awarded according to what side of the bone faced up upon landing. Whoever earned the highest score with the bones got to thump the other players' knuckles. A game of skill (*eto-fvske cakhēcetv*) used a pointed wooden stick thrown from different areas on the body using different grips. When the stick was thrown and it landed upright in the dirt, points were awarded. Then the player progressed to the next level of difficulty.

The adults stressed good and cautious behaviors, warning the children that if they disobeyed, the white person would "take you away, capture

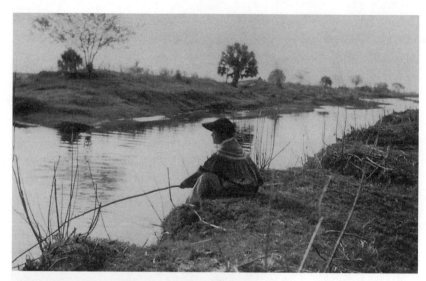

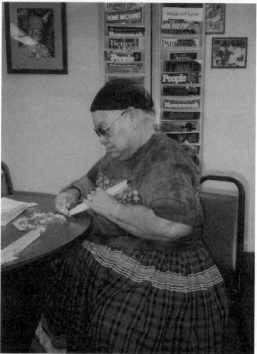

Alice, as a young girl, appears to be fishing on the banks of the Harney Pond Canal at Brighton Reservation in the 1930s. Today she often joins in tribal-sponsored fishing tournaments during Fourth of July celebrations. Photograph from the William D. Boehmer Collection, courtesy of the Department of Anthropology and Genealogy, Seminole Tribe of Florida.

Alice prepares a wooden stick for an old Seminole counting game. Players toss the stick from different starting points on their body, flip it to the ground, and accumulate points when the stick stands up in the sand. Whoever finishes first by flipping the stick from the head is the winner. Photograph courtesy of the Billie Osceola Memorial Library.

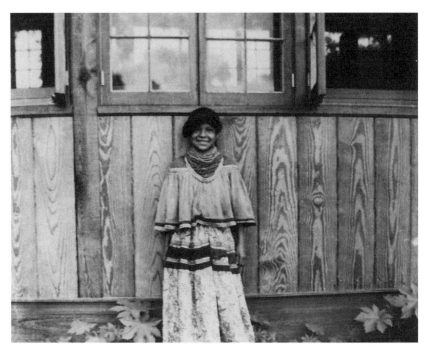

Alice stands before the Brighton Indian Day School in the 1930s. Because she wanted to learn, she defied her mother's warnings against attending school. Photograph from the William D. Boehmer Collection, courtesy of the Department of Anthropology and Genealogy, Seminole Tribe of Florida.

you, or steal you." In addition, the traditional stories told at night reinforced the dangers of leaving the camp. It was against this background of fear and suspicion that Alice's mother refused to let her children attend school.

A day school for the Seminole Indians was established on the reservation in the late 1930s. "Our parents didn't want us to go to school," Alice remembers. "The parents would want us to run away to the hammock when the school bus came." Emma Micco was fearful of what schooling would do to her children. When the bus drove past the camps to provide a ride to school, she would call to her children to hide until the bus was safely down the road. Alice and her brother Jack begged their mother to let them attend school. Jack argued that if the Seminoles could read and write, they would know what they were signing when dealing with the outside world. Their mother finally relented. Learning English would help qualify Alice for her lifelong role as interpreter between the community and the outside world.

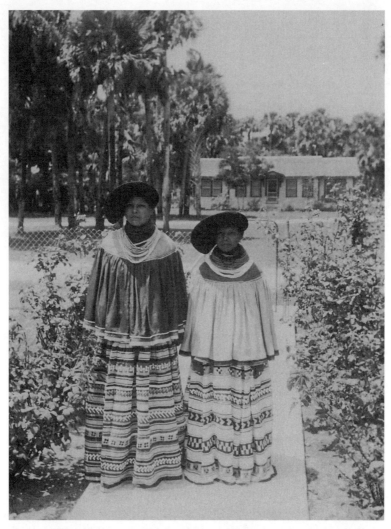

Mary Jo Bowers and Alice stand on the sidewalk in front of the Brighton Indian Day School in the 1930s. Photograph from the William D. Boehmer Collection, courtesy of the Department of Anthropology and Genealogy, Seminole Tribe of Florida.

Alice was the oldest child in the school. "I was about fourteen years old when I started school. Others said I was too old to go to school. My mother heard what they said and told me, 'They don't want you.' I ran away from school one time. The teacher got on the bus and came after us [Alice and her brother Jack]. I quit after the second or third grade." By then, Alice had picked up English. The elders would ask her to talk English for them when they needed to interact with the majority culture. "I did that for my lifetime," she explains. "The Tribe was organized [politically] in 1957. They wanted people to represent Brighton in tribal government. Men folks were rare. People asked me to run because I spoke English. I was the board representative [in 1965–67]." After serving as board representative, Alice decided to further her education: "I needed more education to help the Indian people. We have a lot of school dropouts. In 1973, I went back to school, to night school, for two years. I graduated. I want the children to think, 'If she's old and she graduated, then we can do it, too.' I got all my kids graduated. Now, they have jobs with the Seminole Tribe."

In 1977, Alice spoke to the Seminole youth about education:

[Education] is kind of hard when you talk about [traditional] culture. It depends on who your parents are. I stepped on their toes to go to school. When the school bus came around, they told us to hide in the woods. At school, they wanted us to speak English, but it was hard to do. The teacher didn't want us to speak our language, but we would hide and talk together. We told our families what we learned. It was hard to pick up English. We started listening to our teachers like our parents and talk for our parents. Now we are losing our language. It is hard to get along with your parents if you don't know the language. It will be hard for you to grow up because you don't speak the language.

After I had Carolyn [and Elbert], I went back to night school. Ya'll need to go back to school, get a good education, and help the Seminole Tribe. If you know your language, you can pick it up, then you know what they're saying behind your back.

Alice grew up at a time when the Seminoles hunted game, collected wild foods, or had small gardens. Education had less importance than food. She remembers: "Back then we didn't have many jobs, and [my father] would go out and trap otters, coons, and alligators for us. He would sell the hides for money for the family. He would bring back turtles for us to cook. He would take us wherever he wanted to hunt and we would make a camp and have to stay."

When meat was scarce in the camp, Alice and her sister Cody would go hunting for wild hogs. Alice learned where to find hogs from her mother. Everyone in the camp knew that if Alice and Cody left on horses late in the evening, they would come back with hog meat. Either they would rope the hog and kill it with a knife, or they would herd the animal into water, where they'd capture and drown it. At one time, they killed a hog so big that they had to cut it into two pieces; one half was light enough for each girl to put on the back of her horse to take home.

In the late 1930s, a cattle program was started at the reservation to help provide the Seminoles with a more stable form of subsistence. Alice's father, Charlie Micco, was one of the first trustees of the tribal cattle enter-

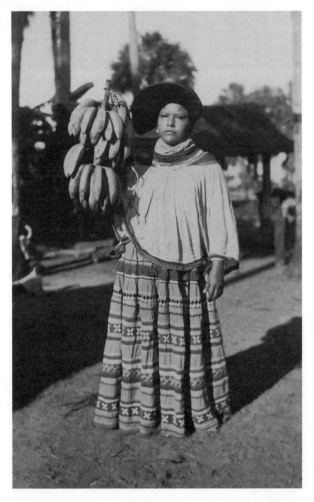

Alice as a young girl holds a bunch of bananas in her family's camp in Glades County (ca. 1930–40). Growing bananas beside the camp gave the family fresh food to eat. Photograph from the William D. Boehmer Collection, courtesy of the Department of Anthropology and Genealogy, Seminole Tribe of Florida.

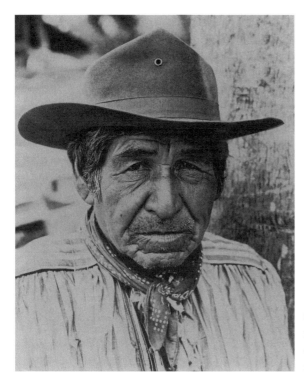

Charlie Micco, Alice's father, was one of the earliest cattle owners in the Tribe.

prise. "[My father] started working with the cattle when they brought the cattle for the Seminole Tribe. He was the one who met the train and brought them back to the reservation. After they learned how to work on the cows, he started to go out to the white people and work for them. When he started working for the white people, he bought a truck for us to ride around. Then he bought a record player for us to play. It was one of the kind that you crank, and when the spring broke, we had to turn it by hand. Then he started to make a cornfield, and he raised good crops one time on the reservation."

Alice's avocation as a go-between for Seminoles in need of traditional medicine and the Indian doctors began simply with learning to identify the herbs used. Traditional learning is a matter of observation and doing. There was no purposeful teaching of the correct botanicals to use, but a slow, natural socialization into the role. Alice's mother would call to her, "Come with me." They would walk through the woods, sometimes for quite a distance, gathering and carrying the plants.

In much the same way Alice taught me about herbs, her mother would point to the plants she needed and give instructions. For example, she might say, "Bring me *tolv*. Get it from the east side." Through repeated

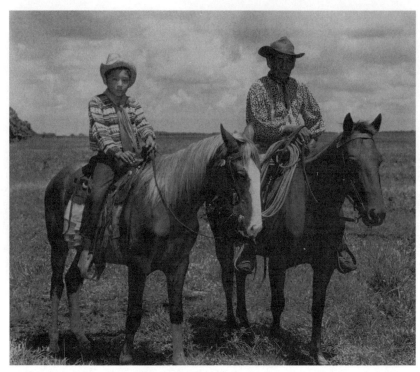

Charlie Micco and his grandson Fred Smith are pictured on their horses when they take a break from rounding up their cattle (ca. 1930s–1940s).

trips into the woods to collect the ingredients for each specific medicine, Alice learned to identify every plant by its Creek name. She became a keen observer of place and habitat of the medicine, almost intuitively knowing what kind of area to look in and in what season. Her sister Leona learned in the same manner. If, after the death of her mother, Alice had a question about the location or identification of a specific herb, she would call her sister Leona for advice.

As a young woman, Alice also learned Mikasuki, the other language of the Seminoles, so she could talk with a Miccosukee friend of hers. This friend, Mary Tiger, knew no Creek (Alice's language), and Alice knew no Mikasuki (Mary's language). When they worked together on a tomato farm, Alice learned Mary's language by talking to her and asking her what the names for different things were. Both girls asked each other until they learned each other's language.

Following Seminole tradition, when Alice married Bob Snow, a member of the Panther clan, on August 4, 1948, it was their mothers who arranged the marriage. Initially, the couple lived in Alice's family camp. By the time Alice had her youngest daughter, Salina, she and Bob were living in a small, enclosed chickee with a tin roof that they had made. In the 1960s, they moved into a HUD-sponsored concrete-block house in the center of the community; Alice still lives in that house today. Bob took care of medicine for Indian doctors at the Green Corn Dance. He collected herbs for the bundles, which only men were allowed to do. Bob also worked for the Lykes Brothers company, picking tomatoes and driving a dump truck. In 1985, he was a cook at Alice's Restaurant, a reservation café, when he was killed in a car accident early one foggy morning on the way to work.

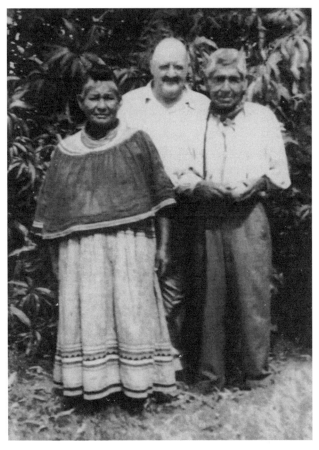

Emma and Charlie Micco pose with Jack Devane (*center*) in this rare photo of Alice's mother and father together. Devane was a friend to the Indians and brought treats at Christmastime. The photograph was taken during the 1930s.

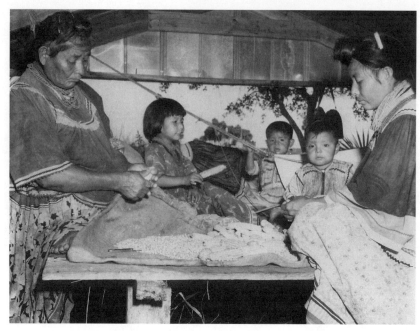

Emma Micco and Leona Micco Smith shell corn in their chickee while Emma's grandchildren Nellie Smith, Rufus Tiger, and Jack Smith, Jr., watch. Corn is prepared and ground to cook into the traditional drink, *sofkee*.

Alice had five children: Jenny, Smawley, twins Elbert and Carolyn, and Salina. The first, Jenny, was born when Alice was just eighteen. She describes how *tolv* was used in connection with Jenny's birth: "I had Jenny in the hospital. Before I left the hospital, they rubbed *tolv* on my body. They burned the leaves in the car, put it inside the car. They went around the car four times with the burnt leaves and waved burnt leaves near both sides of the face and forehead and put it on Jenny. When I brought her home, they also fixed a bundle of *tolv*, treated it, and brought it to her and rubbed it on her. Sometimes we put [a bundle] on the swing (*estuce 'sem vholasketv*).[1]

Alice used baby medicine when she had all her children. The treatments were accompanied by restrictions. Restrictions are similar to the instructions that come with Western prescriptions—stating what is appropriate to ingest with the medicine. If the restrictions are not followed, the medicine is rendered ineffective or sometimes misfortune may befall the Indian doctor. Alice explains her restrictions after each birth and the ritual that accompanies birth:

If you nurse the baby, you are the one that gets on restriction. The baby's not able to eat anyway. No backbones, inside [innards], and turkey, mudfish, and *holakwv* [soft-shell turtle]. Right after four days, we have to start eating with the family again. I could have slept outside with the baby, too. My mother could sleep with me, but I had [the baby] in the hospital.

I used the Indian medicine before I left the hospital. When we bring [the baby] back, we cross over canals and they told me I have to call her all the time till we get home. I called, "*Wakoce vta, wakoce vta.*"[2] I called her name or her little spirit. If I don't, the little spirit, the one she's got, would be left behind if I didn't call her all the time. She would be crying all night, crying all the time. She told me I have to call her until I get home.

We didn't have an Indian name when we got out of the hospital, so we had to call her by her English name. She was given an English

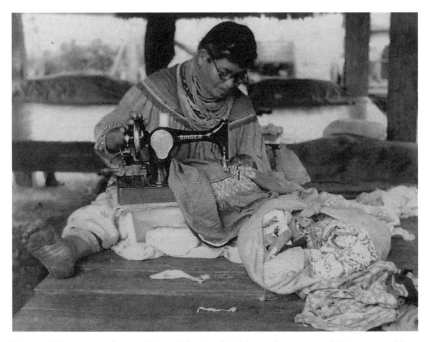

Emma Micco sews the traditional Seminole skirt on her manual Singer machine. Her daughter Alice continues to sew traditional clothes today for her children and for grandchildren's princess contests, for festival dress contests, and to sell to friends and tourists for extra income.

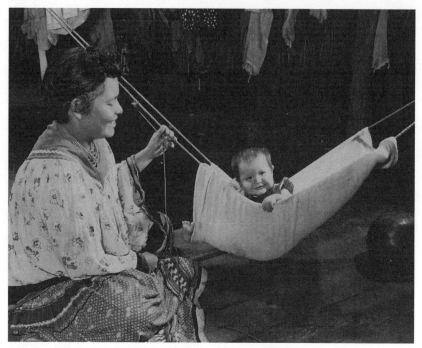

This photo accompanied Louis Capron's article on the Seminoles that appeared in *National Geographic* in 1956. Alice is shown swinging her baby Smawley (ca. 1952) in the cleverly designed traditional baby rocker and cradle strung between posts of her chickee home. Photograph by David S. Boyer, courtesy of the NGS Image Collection.

name after a white person I worked on the farm with in town. The woman had asked me to name it after her.

We didn't give Indian names until we brought them home, and we have to find an old lady to ask her to give her a regular name. You have to tell her ahead of time so she can think it over. Then she comes over and gives the name. I found an old lady to give her a Creek name. She came over. She could tell ahead and gave her the name *Vhecoke*, which means "it looks forward." She has to hold it and name it. She gives it back, and then you have to call her name four times.

After I got home [from the hospital], I had to stay in a separate little chickee and could see the family from the chickee. My chickee was next to where the family slept. Women came to see me, but man folks could not see us for four days.

Two or three weeks later after I had the baby, I go and take a bath, wash all my clothes, and move into my husband's chickee. He built the chickee in my mother's camp. Before I can eat with the family again, I have to get treated with *tolv* in water. This was so I won't get sick.

We would make one whole gallon can. That's what we used to mix the medicine with. He treated it one time, and I just have to give her the bath then give it back to him again after four times. *Heles-here* was in it. *Tolv* and, like, *pvrko, coloswuce, cafvknv, ue-heleswv, akwanv,* and *lucv-huehkv.*

My father treated my kids. He gave them the *vtelokuce* after I had those babies. Little small babies when they are born, they're not real humans, and they call that *vtelokuce.* They have to fix that, and they have to give a bath for her four times in the morning. We have to go

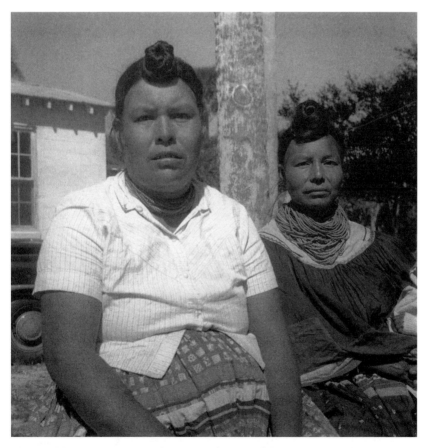

Alice and her sister Leona in the 1950s. Photograph by Irvin M. Peithmann, courtesy of the Florida State Archives.

through that *sofkee, afkoce hvtke,* and all that stuff. That's the way they make the human a person. I did that for Jenny, Salina, all of my children.

Alice says that "for the easier treatments, many women are doctors. Some old ladies are doctors, too." She considers herself to be "a little bit" *heles hayv,* or Indian doctor, because she specializes in collecting the herbs and acting as a go-between for tribal members and the Indian doctors. She is particularly important for being the "legs" of elders who are not mobile enough to collect the herbs and transport them to the Indian doctor for treatment.

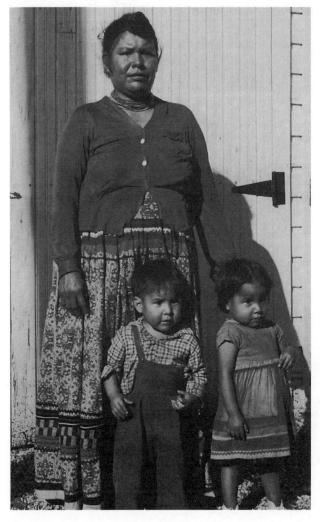

Alice stands before a barn with her twin children, Elbert and Carolyn (ca. 1957). Photograph from the Peithmann Collection, courtesy of the Florida State Archives.

Alice has been around Indian medicine throughout her life. Her father fixed the medicine and gave treatments, while her mother collected the herbs for the medicine. "My dad knew other kinds of medicine, like treatment for the pain and all that stuff. We didn't have shoes in that time, and we had a lot of sores on our feet. My dad fixed the medicine for that too. He also fixed baby treatment for us, too. When my son [Jim] died,[3] when I had another one, he gave a treatment for four months, one at a time for each month. He gave it to the baby so that this baby would survive."

Alice describes the early training she received from her mother:

The first time I started collecting for the Indian medicine was when my—I call him Grampa [Calo Harjo, her mother's mother's brother]—died. At that time my mother collected the medicine. She told me what it was used for. I just watched how she collected the medicine in the woods. I didn't ask her questions, but she told me what the things were for. She told me the names, and back then she had a lot of them to collect. She collected *tolv* first. That's the one we're using now, but I'm pretty sure they also used water oak and pine trees and maple and cedar.

She had a lot of different material to take to the doctor. She had more materials than we use today. She had ones that we use to make a dress, ones with flowers on it. And ones that had stripes, too. She gave the material to the medicine man with knives, an ax—whatever he asked for. Most times a hog, too. The hog had to be around the medicine too, when they fixed it. That's as far as I remember.

When my grampa Calo Harjo died, they laid him out. He died in the morning. They told us he died, and they didn't want us to go around the dead body. And they just put us in another chickee. We had to sit down and sit still. We were not supposed to watch where they were moving the body or anything. Just a few people can see that body when they move it. We didn't have caskets back them. They said they built a little ol' box and put it on top of the ground. They took the body into the woods outside of the yard. After they put the body in the woods, they had to build a little fire beside him. When they come back, we were not supposed to see those people, the ones that were burying the body. The next day they had to go back and build the fire again for him. They do it like that for four days.

We just sat there for four days, no playing around. We couldn't change our clothes. We didn't have to comb our hair. They didn't want us to look where the sun goes down. We are supposed to face the east all the time. The medicine was kept by the fire on the west side. We had to drink it and face east. We were not supposed to carry the medicine away from the fire. The restrictions were the same as they are today. And they were strict, too. They didn't want us to break anything but stick with it for four months. Even they didn't want us to go to town or spend the money or touch the money for four days. We could get up and play again after four days.

They just put the body out in the woods and left it out there. But I ran into it one time when I was riding a horse. It was a little box about the same size as the person. They had two tree limbs at the end standing that were crossed, but when I saw it that cross had fallen down in. I didn't look too close. As soon as I saw it, I turned the horse around. I was about thirteen or fourteen at the time.

My mother was the one who collected the medicine and made us use it. She was the one who gathered it up, but my daddy fixed it. He sat with the medicine by the fire and sang and blew in it. I mean, it's a long song [for death medicine] too. They have to do it four times each day for four days.

Nowadays, according to Alice, there is more of a mix of Western and Indian medicine:

We go to the clinic and get pills. We used to get shots, but today we get pills. It sometimes helps and sometimes it doesn't. Sometimes you get some herbs and go to the Indian doctor. Or you do both. If you go to a white doctor, sometimes you won't be cured. Sometimes the Indian doctor works.

Alice's belief in the medicine remains a central part of her life today, although after losing an infant at birth she turned from her native religion and its major ceremony, the Green Corn Dance, to Christianity. Since then, she has been an active participant in the congregation of the First Indian Baptist Church on the Brighton Reservation. Being Baptist has changed some of Alice's behavior. For example, she has not drunk alcohol for more than thirty years because the church views drinking as contrary to Christian witness. Nevertheless, she has always treated the Green Corn Dance with respect and encourages others to do the same because "this is our religion." She contrasts the way this ceremony is conducted today with practices of the past: "When they have the Green Corn Dance (*eshvyvtketv*), it's not the way it used to be long ago. My mother told me it was sacred and there was no drinking. There used to be a lot of older people teaching those things. Now you don't have no older people. Last year [1997] was the

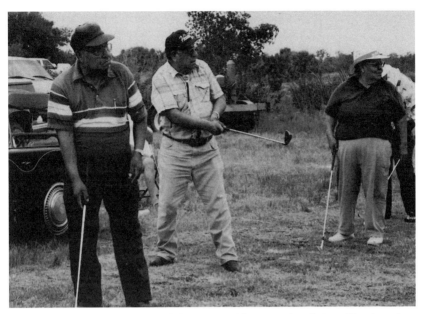

Jack Micco, Howard Micco, and their sister Alice practice their golf swings in a Fourth of July celebration on the reservation. The three also enjoy bowling and horseshoes. Photograph courtesy of the *Seminole Tribune.*

worse one [for losing elders]. [During the ceremony] you were playing like at school. The men folks pushed the women down. A long time ago when fasting day came, women were fasting too—even the little children, too, until after the feather dance (*fus-hesse 'sopvnkv*). We did it, but not real fasting—we drank water, beer, or wine."

Like many other Seminoles, Alice loves to travel, driving long distances to do missionary work for her church. Because of her frequent travel to faraway places such as North Dakota and New Mexico, Alice has friends throughout the nation. My first road trip with Alice was to Davie, Oklahoma, to attend Indian Falls Creek, an annual conference in which Native American Baptists from all over the United States gather for a week of worship and Bible study. She knew the way to Davie without a map. When it was my turn to drive, I had only to wait for her command, "Turn here."

Before the start of Indian Falls Creek, we visited a dry goods store in Wewoka, Oklahoma. As we were browsing through the material on a table, a man and woman approached, saying, "Why, Alice Snow! How are you doing?" They had remembered Alice from her former trips. This was the first of many adventures where we ran into people who remembered

Alice's Seminole Rules of Life

You have to teach your children what the elders taught us: how to get married, how to comb your hair, and how to behave when kinfolk die.

Your eyes reveal the end of the world. You can see the reading in your eyes, and it will be the end of your culture. *Meheleskel* will come down and see the reading in your eyes.

When visitors come to our camp, we show respect. We see them coming from far off and walk to meet them. We would say to the young children, "Go get some cold water, they're going to be thirsty." We give them cold water to drink. We put coffee on the fire. We have no doors, so we couldn't ask them to come in. We would have food on the table and ask them to eat before they leave. Today, people meet you at the door and say, "What do you want?" They should invite them in like we learned.

When you go to someone's home, sit down and don't move around or touch anything. When we [the children] stayed at home, the seven brothers and sisters played together, but not in someone else's camp.

When eating, the children eat last.

When children did wrong, we would get a whipping. Also, our uncle or grandpa scratched us to make us behave.[4]

Whatever someone says to you, don't get mad, just go. It will come back to them later.

When you are pregnant, don't watch monkeys. Babies are like monkeys and won't behave.

Alice. When she goes to these places, she usually inquires about other Indian doctors so that she can find medicine unavailable in South Florida and learn about new treatments.

Alice has always been an independent person, whether venturing outside her culture or boldly challenging her mother's decision that she should not attend school. Her personality has taken her in interesting directions. In addition to serving as board representative for the Brighton community, she has worked as a chickee builder, fence contractor, bus driver, mower, field hand, mental health and alcohol counselor for the Indian medicine program, café owner and operator, palmetto fan collector, and, most recently, as Head Start and nursery granny. She has sold huckleberries, guavas, palmetto buds, beadwork, tomahawks, frog legs, Indian burgers, pumpkin bread, and Seminole patchwork dresses, jackets, and vests to help make ends meet.

However, of all Alice's jobs, helping her people retain their culture in a rapidly changing world remains the closest to her heart. She is concerned about the loss of tradition and traditional values, such as showing respect toward the elderly. She identifies additional factors that are threatening the Seminole way of life: "I don't know how long the Tribe will last. We are losing Indians to mixed blood, one-quarter ancestry. We are also losing the Indians to alcohol. We are also losing them because they don't get a college education."

This handbook of Seminole herbs and their uses, the compendium of a lifetime's knowledge and practice in herbal medicine, is part of Alice's solution to the problem of disappearing religious and social values. Her goal is to help Seminoles hold on to their past while living in the present and moving toward the future.

II

Alice's Handbook
of Seminole Medicine

5

Treatments

◆◆◆◆◆◆◆◆◆◆◆◆◆◆◆◆◆◆◆

Cool Medicine

Kv·svp·pe he·les·wv
(Ka·baa·le a·yek·che)

Herbs to Collect

Creek name	Mikasuki name	English common name
1. *to·lv*	*too·le*	bay
2. *ak·wa·nv*	*o·ke·bak·she*	willow
3. *he·to·tv·pe*	*ep·taa·pe*	frost weed
4. *ue-he·les·wv*	*yah·ka·ka-yek·che*	lizard's tail

How to Use the Medicine

Cool medicine is used when someone has an operation. Mix ingredients in water and take them to doctor to be treated. When the medicine is fixed, the people have to drink it four times, facing east, and use it on their bodies, especially where they were cut.

Take red material or red and white material, depending on the medicine man.

Restrictions *(e·mv·seh·kv; e·ma·ye·pee·ke)*

· No hot foods.
· No hot coffee (warm is okay).
· No going out of house (current restriction of some doctors, but not all).

67

In the past, the restrictions applied for four days, but now they are just done for two days.

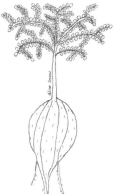

Treatment for Hysterectomy

Cos·tak·hu·te en·lvf·ho·yat

Herbs to Collect

Creek name	Mikasuki name	English common name
1. *to·lv*	*too·le*	bay
2. *ak·wa·nv*	*o·ke·bak·she*	willow
3. *he·les·hvt·ke*	*a·yek·che·hvt·ke*	ginseng
4. *ue·he·les·wv*	*yah·ka·ka·yek·che*	lizard's tail

If you need a stronger medicine, you need to get the bay leaves first, then willow (cold medicine) and lizard's tail plant. When you put these together, they will make a stronger medicine.

How to Use the Medicine

This Indian medicine is taken after a hysterectomy operation. It is like cold medicine. It is used for healing the cut and for pain relief. All of the above ingredients are mixed with ginseng root in water. The mixture is then taken to an Indian doctor to be treated. He or she will tell you how to use it. The doctor may tell you to drink some medicine and put it on the cut or where the pain is located four times a day or as many times as you want to use it. When using the medicine, do not eat or drink really hot things, but wait until the food or drink is lukewarm before consuming it. Do this for two to four days. Do not pick up heavy things for four days.

The medicine man should receive four colors of material. Bring the medicine man four yards each of red, black, white, and yellow. These colors are known as the medicine colors.

Restrictions (four months)

· No smoking.
· No alcohol.
· No backbones.
· No insides (innards—chitlins, liver, etc.).
· No hot foods or drink.
· Do not hold a little baby for eight days.

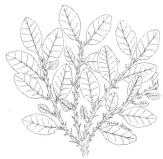

Pain Treatment

Nok·kat en·he·les·ha·ye·tv
(No·kaa·cheh·che e·ma·yek·cho·mee·ke)

Herbs to Collect

Creek name	Mikasuki name	English common name
1. *he·les-hvt·ke*	*a·yek·che-hat·ke*	ginseng

A lot of people use different things for pain, but I use *heles-hvtke,* or ginseng root. Use four little pieces of the roots. Put water in a jar the size of a pop bottle. Leave room in the jar for the doctor to blow in it. Add the scrapings or small pieces of the *heles-hvtke* to the jar. Take the jar to the doctor for treatment.

Take four yards of white material to the doctor.

How to Use the Medicine

Use the medicine by putting it on the place where it hurts, drinking a little (sipping) or licking it with the ring finger four times. The doctor will tell you that if the pain does not go away, leave a small amount of medicine in the bottle and bring it back to him or her. The doctor will add more water and treat it again. Use the medicine again until the pain goes away.

Restriction (four days)

· Do not eat meat that has blood clots in it.

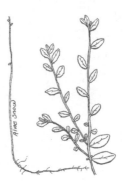

A Treatment for a Lot of Pain

Herbs to Collect

Creek name	Mikasuki name	English common name
1. *he·les-hvt·ke*	*a·yek·che-hat·ke*	ginseng
2. *to·lv*	*too·le*	bay

One of the old Indian doctors used this treatment. He liked to ask more about the nature of the pain and where it is located. This is the best and strongest medicine. It requires four yards of red material and $100. The doctor likes to put a lot of restrictions with this medicine.

How to Use the Medicine

When you use the medicine, you have to eat supper first, then use it two times before you go to sleep and two more times the next morning.

Restriction (until medicine is used up)

· Do not eat salt. Before you use salt, get a little bag of dry willow bark, mix it with water, and take a bath with it first. Put the liquid where the pain exists.

Restrictions (four months)

· No insides (innards).
· No liver.
· No backbone.
· No liver cheese.
· No hog's head cheese.
· No chitlins.

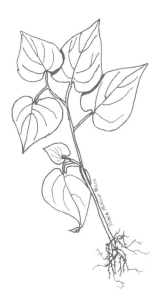

Ear Treatment

Hvc·ko-nok·kat en·he·les-ha·ye·tv
(Hak·cho·be-no·kaa·che·ka e·ma·yek·cho·mee·ke)

How to Use the Medicine

The person must come to the doctor and ask for the treatment for the ear that hurts. The doctor will make the treatment if the person brings old material. It does not have to be usable but should be ragged. The doctor asks the person for the material.

The doctor uses a pipe handle or straw. He or she asks the patient which side is hurt and begins the treatment on the opposite side by blowing gently through the pipe handle four times. The doctor sings a song at this time, then waits five minutes and blows in the other side four times. The doctor does this four times. After the doctor is finished, he or she picks up the material and throws it away. If the ear is infected, the pain won't go away and the person goes to the clinic doctor. He says after that, "If it still hurts, let me know."

Restriction (four months)

· Don't eat the meat from any animal's head like hog's head cheese.

Treatment for Stroke

E·na ē·lat en·he·les·ha·ye·tv
(Ak·ne e·mel·la·ka em a·yek·cho·mee·ke)

Herbs to Collect

Creek name	Mikasuki name	English common name
1. *to·lv*	*too·le*	bay
2. *ue·he·les·wv*	*yah·ka·ka·yek·che*	lizard's tail
3. *ak·wa·nv*	*o·ke·bak·she*	willow
4. *he·to·tv·pe*	*ep·taa·pe*	frost weed
5. *he·fe·pe nēr·kv*	*he·fe·pe ee·le*	bottle gourd seeds
6. *tot·kv cok·hes·se*	*ee·te choos·ke*	ground moss
7. *ē·kv·nv cok·hes·se*	*yak·ne choos·ke*	spiked sedge
8. *pas·sv*	*pa·she*	button snakeroot

How to Use the Medicine

Use the medicine cold. Use it at night. Drink a little bit with the tip of the fingers and tongue, and take a bath in the morning with it for four mornings. After the night, don't eat until after you take it in the morning.

Restrictions

· Don't touch a knife or share anything for one day.
· Don't walk around in the rain for four days.
· Don't look at anything that died—people or animals—or their things for eight days.
· For four months, do not eat insides or backbones.
· Eat alone for four months.

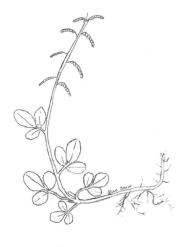

Treatment for a Person Who Blacks Out or Is Short of Breath

Es·te ker·re·kot ha·ke⁻·pvt en·he·les-ha·ye·tv
(Es·te he·sa·ke·tv en·ko·cok·nat en·he·les-ha·ye·tv)

Herbs to Collect

Creek name	Mikasuki name	English common name
1. *he·les-hvt·ke*	*a·yek·che-hat·ke*	ginseng

How to Use the Medicine

An old Indian doctor told me that when a person blacks out or is short of breath, you need to take four little pieces of *heles-hvtke* and put them in water. Get the ginseng treated by a doctor. If the doctor asks you to put the ginseng in water, then you have to drink it. But if the doctor treats it dry, he may place the medicine under the tongue of a person who has fainted. Let the person lie there. Sometimes they come out of it. You need ginseng root with you at all times because usually the doctor will ask you if you have any. A lot of people have it on hand. Sometimes I have it with me in case someone faints at a funeral, can hardly breathe, or gets weak. If a doctor is available, he or she can treat the person right there. In exchange for treatment, you will always need to give the doctor white material.

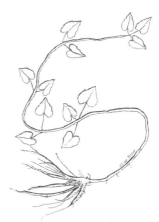

Treatment for a Speeding Heart

E·fē·ke em·pvf·nan he·les-ha·ye·tv

Herbs to Collect

Creek name	Mikasuki name	English common name
1. *he·les-hvt·ke*	*a·yek·che-hat·ke*	ginseng

How to Use the Medicine

I went to the doctor and asked him what he could do for that kind of treatment. He said to put a little piece of ginseng root in water, and he would fix it. I added some extra *heles-hvtke* to make it stronger. Use it four days. When you use it, face east. Pass the liquid around your head four times clockwise. Drink four swallows. Put some medicine in your hand and rub it around your chest four times. Bring four yards of white material to the doctor.

Restriction (four months)

• Do not eat heart.

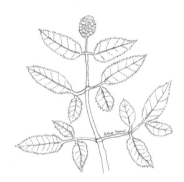

Treatment for Someone Who Has Been Ill for a Long Time and Is Afraid to Walk

Herbs to Collect

Creek name	Mikasuki name	English common name
1. *to·lv*	*too·le*	bay
2. *ak·wa·nv*	*o·ke·bak·she*	willow (at least one strip of the bark must be one foot long)
3. *lu·cv-hueh·kv en·hom·pe·tv*	*a·paa·ho·she em·em·pee·ke*	gopher apple
4. *v·ce os·tet*	*ash·pe shee·taa·ken*	four pieces of corn

How to Use the Medicine

Get herbs—bay, willow, gopher turtle food, and four pieces of corn. Put them together and mix with water in a gallon jar. Take this to the Indian doctor and have it treated. The medicine must be kept cold.

When you get the treatment back from the doctor, put the medicine on your hips and legs. Take a one-foot strip of bark of the willow plant from the jar and whip the hips and legs easily.

There are no food restrictions with this medicine because the body is already weak.

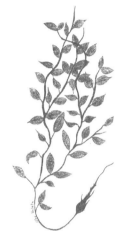

Treatment If You Like to Sleep All the Time

Herbs to Collect

Creek name	Mikasuki name	English common name
1. *to·lv*	*too·le*	bay
2. *hel·es-he·re*	*a·yek·che-hee·le*	downy milk pea
3. *he·fe·pe nēr·kv*	*he·fe·pe ee·le*	bottle gourd seeds
4. *ue-he·les·wv*	*yah·ka·ka-yek·che*	lizard's tail

How to Use the Medicine

Mix the herbs with water and take them to the doctor and let the doctor fix them. Give the doctor a gift of the following:
· four yards of black and four yards of white material;
· a knife;
· a black chicken (if no black chicken is available, you may substitute a chicken you buy in the store);
· four big shotgun shells;
· a spool of white thread;
· black or white beads (if the person being treated is a woman) or a black or white handkerchief (if the person being treated is a man).

If you don't have all that, you may give money. The amount is up to you.

The doctor will treat some grits and give it to you. Before taking the medicine, prepare the grits. Make it into *osafke hvtke* (thin white grits).

Early in the morning before you have had food, take a bath with the medicine that is in the water. Wait a little bit. Bathe with it again until you have repeated it for four times. After the bath, use your ring finger to dip into the *osafke hvtke* and lick the finger. Do that four times.

After that, put the *osafke* on your body: on your hands, face, and legs but never on your belly. What's left you have to eat. After you use the *osafke*, you can eat anything but the things that are restricted.

Restrictions (four months)

· No young deer.
· No turkey.
· No backbones.
· No insides.
· No cigarettes.
· No alcohol.
· No soft-shell turtle.
· No mudfish.

Restrictions (eight days)

· Don't let a dog touch you.
· Don't take a bath in open water, a canal, or the ocean.
· Don't go out in the rain.
· Don't hold a baby.

When you use this treatment, it makes you feel good. If you get tired easily, it will help you. The same treatment is for pain and sleeping all the time.

I went to the doctor and told him that I had a pain on my hand on the little finger and that I sometimes get headaches. He said that might come from the heart and that he was going to treat it. He said to get the *ueheleswv* (lizard's tail plant) and rub the area with it. He said to pour the medicine on my head. After taking the medicine, you get really sleepy, but you will not go to sleep until after 12 noon. Then you can sleep.

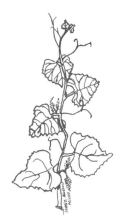

Mixed Medicine Treatment

V·te·lo·ku·ce he·les·wv

Herbs to Collect

Creek name	Mikasuki name	English common name
1. *to·lv*	*too·le*	bay
2. *ue–he·les·wv*	*yah·ka·ka–yek·che*	lizard's tail plant
3. *ak·wa·nv*	*o·ke·bak·she*	willow
4. *pvr·ko*	*baɫ·be*	wild grapes
5. *ca·fvk·nv*	*o·la·ke*	huckleberry
6. *he·to·tv·pe*	*ep·taa·pe*	frost weed

How to Use the Medicine

This treatment puts all kinds of herbs together and mixes them. Its name, *vtelokuce,* means "something that you bring all together," like something that is spilled and you try to get it all together. It is used when you don't want a lot of restrictions. More people can use it. It is used for the person who is weak and wants to sleep all the time and doesn't want to do anything. That person has to take a bath with it and drink it to cure the sickness.

Treatment for Not Being Able to Sleep When You Want, for Worry, and for Bad Dreams

Herbs to Collect

Creek name	Mikasuki name	English common name
1. *to·lv*	*too·le*	bay

Get a lot of *tolv* leaves and have the doctor treat them. If you are dreaming about people who are already dead, use it. The doctor says we need to clear the road for the bad spirit.

How to Use the Medicine

After the doctor has fixed the *tolv*, face east. Hold a bit of it and rub it on your body all over. Crush it in your hands and smell it. Do not turn left after using it. If you have to turn left, then turn right in a circle to get to the position. Next put a bundle of it under your pillow and sleep.

If you have heard something moving around in the house, you can burn *tolv* inside the house. Burning gets rid of the thing that was moving around. It provides protection.

There are no restrictions with this treatment. If you need more *tolv*, you can get some fresh leaves and add them to the treated ones and the treatment will continue to be effective.

Treatment for Bad Dreams

He·re·ko e·stv·pue·cv en·he·les·wv

Herbs to Collect

Creek name	Mikasuki name	English common name
First kind		
1. *to·lv*	*too·le*	bay
2. *he·les-he·re*	*a·yek·che-hee·le*	downy milk pea
3. *'stv·lok·pu·ce*		beggar's lice
4. *he·fe·pe-nēr·kv*	*he·fe·pe ee·le*	bottle gourd seeds
Second kind		
1. *to·lv*	*too·le*	bay
2. *he·les-he·re*	*a·yek·che-hee·le*	downy milk pea
3. *'stv·lok·pu·ce*		beggar's lice
4. *he·fe·pe-nēr·kv*	*he·fe·pe ee·le*	bottle gourd seeds

5. *ue-he·les·wv*	*yah·ka·ka·yek·che*	lizard's tail
6. *ak·wa·nv*	*o·ke·bak·she*	willow
7. *lu·cv-hueh·ka en·hom·pe·tv*	*a·paa·ho·she em·em·pee·ke*	gopher apple

When you have a bad dream about someone and you want to protect him or her, use this medicine. Usually the Indian doctor wants to know what the dream was about. It took the Indian doctor over an hour to fix the medicine in a one-gallon jug.

Give the Indian doctor four yards of black material, four gun shells, one spool of white thread, a knife, beads, handkerchief, and sometimes a chicken.

The material and items given to the Indian doctor are supposed to be given away to someone in a different clan, but many doctors give the material to their wives to sew designs.

How to Use the Medicine

Find a big pot to put the medicine in. Use it early in the morning before you eat. If the medicine is for your children, the oldest child takes it first, then the next according to descending age. Take a bath with it and drink a little bit, in four swallows. Pour it over the body. When you finish with the youngest, start over with the oldest. Do this four times. After the kids use this four times each, then the person who had the dream uses it up.

Restrictions (four days)

· Don't watch TV shows that show violence.
· Don't get mad at a dog.
· Don't touch a knife for one day.

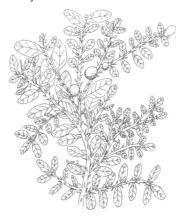

Treatment for Monkey Sickness

Wot·ko-es·te nok·ke·tv ha·yv

Herbs to Collect

Creek name	Mikasuki name	English common name
1. *to·lv*	*too·le*	bay
2. *ak·wa·nv*	*o·ke·bak·she*	willow

Monkey sickness occurs when monkeys make you sick and you begin acting like a monkey. To act like a monkey means you touch your skin with your fingers at different places repeatedly, like monkeys pick at their fur and then look at the tips of their fingers or move them to their nose or mouth.

Put the *tolv* and *akwanv* in water in a bottle and take them to the doctor to be fixed. The medicine requires a live animal and four yards of material. If the doctor has no place to keep a live animal such as a cow, horse, or hog, then give a gift of $100 instead.

How to Use the Medicine

The medicine is used cold. It is used two times in the afternoon after supper and then again two times in the morning. Each time, it is drunk four times (eight altogether). What is left in the morning is used to take a bath, until it is used up. Put it on the face, arms, and legs.

Restrictions (until medicine is used up)

· No salt; the person can get another medicine of just *akwanv* so the person can use salt.

Restrictions (four months)

· Don't get close to monkeys, elephants, cats, tigers, or coons.
· Don't look at the body of a person who has recently died; even when pictures of the person come on TV, don't look at them.

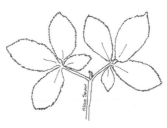

Plants and Their Properties

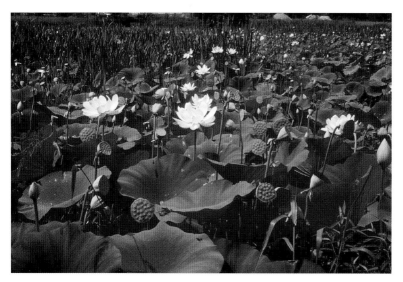

1. *Akkotorkv*   Lotus   *Nelumbo lutea*

You can find this plant in the water. It has big round leaves, yellow flowers, and a big green seedpod. When the pod turns brown or is dried out, we get the seeds out and crack them. The white meat part is good to eat, and in the center are little green things, which I was told are good for whooping cough. Sometimes the seeds fall out of the pod, and we have to look under the water for them. There aren't many of these plants any more because the white people take them out by the trailer full and take them up north and sell them. They use them for flower arrangements. (Slide by W. S. Judd.)

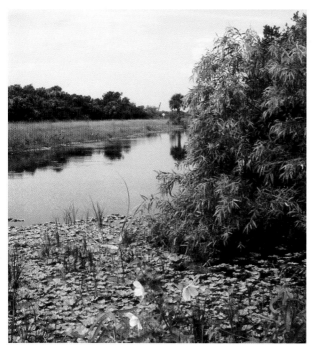

2. *Akwanv*   Willow   *Salix carolinia*

Akwanv is found along canals or near wet ground. It looks like a bush but has rough bark. It has long shiny leaves with white flowers. In the winter, the branches are bare, and the bark is hard to peel. It is used for most everything. The roots are best to use, but if you can't get the roots get the bark. Gather the bark on the east side of the plant. I usually take along an ax or knife and peel it off in strips. When the leaves are green and lush, in July, the bark is easy to peel. Use more to make the medicine stronger or taste good. The more you use, the redder the water of the medicine becomes.

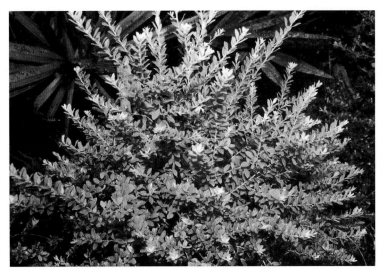

3. *Cafaknv* Huckleberry, blueberry *Vaccinium darrowii* Camp.

Cafaknv grows in open, dry areas in conjunction with pine trees. It can be found everywhere in dry areas. At first I didn't know it was used for medicine. As a child, I would pick the berries and sell them. We used to eat them, too. There are three different kinds of *cafaknv*. *Cafaknv lvstuce* has dark shiny leaves; it is the one we use most. *Cafaknv sopakhvtke* has gray or silver green leaves with gray berries. The last is *copo-peleksv*, which is taller than *cafaknv lvstuce*, growing on one stem with wider leaves. The berries are bigger and have big seeds. This one is used for pies and jellies. We ate and sold all varieties. When collecting *cafaknv* for medicine, get one good-sized plant with the roots. Check with the doctor to find out what parts to get because the parts used vary with the treatment.

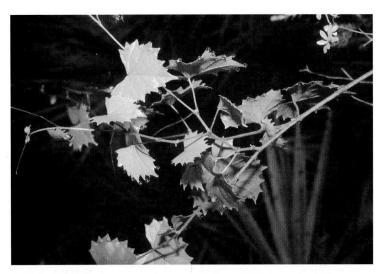

4. *Culoswuce* Little muscadine grape or southern fox grape *Cissus munsoniana* Simpson

You can find this plant anywhere—around the road, on the oak trees, on the fences in a damp area. It crawls to the top of a tree. The green leaves have little points on them and ragged edges and are almost heart shaped. The vine has little black fruit. It has tendrils, which it uses for support for climbing. Collect about a foot or two of the growing end of the vine. If you have to make a lot for death medicine (about five gallons or more), collect one piece about a yard long. Cut it into little pieces to put in water. Just get the vines and leaves. It is used for most everything—cold medicine, death medicine.

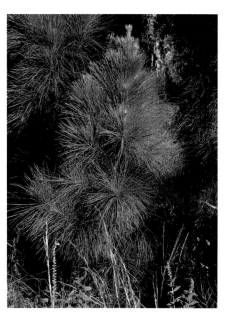

5. *Cule* Slash pine *Pinus caribaea* Morelet
Cule is easy to find because it grows all over. The tree is tall with long needles. For medicine, collect the tip of the growing end. Usually get four four-inch pieces. Sometimes you are asked to get the bark. When used in a woman's treatment, just the forked stem of the pine branch is used. For use on sores, crush *cule* with a hammer, put it in water, add *vtakrv-lvste* (dog fennel), and boil. Wash the sores to clean them really well. This remedy does not need to be treated by a doctor.

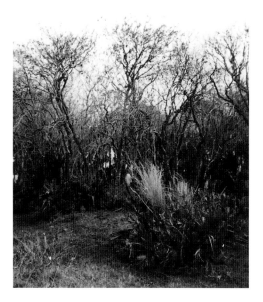

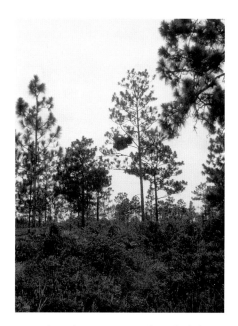

6. *Este lopockuce emeto* "Where the little people live" Bundles of needles of *Pinus caribaea* Morelet
Este lopockuce emeto literally means "where the little people live." Look for a thick bundle of pine needles on the limb of a pine tree. It is hard to find. If the bundle is not too high when you collect it, you can pull it down or use a stick to break it off, but catch it when it falls so it won't touch the ground. If it touches the ground, you have to get another one. (Every medicine that falls on the ground must be left where it fell.) If you are not able to reach the bundle, just get the bark off the tree. This medicine is used when a person who's sick sees a lot of little people around him or her. After the bundle is treated and given, the sick person won't see them any more. It keeps them away. The people tell me that there are a lot of little people around, but we don't see them except when we are sick. This treatment is not used very much.

7. *Eto-hvtkv* Carolina ash *Fraxinus caroliniana* Miller
Eto-hvtkv is found in low, wet, swampy areas, usually as a cluster of trees. It gets its name, "white tree," from the appearance of the underside of the branches. The tree has small white flowers. It is used for a lot of different medicines, like women's medicine. For that, you collect the fork of the branch. Limbs or bark are usually used.

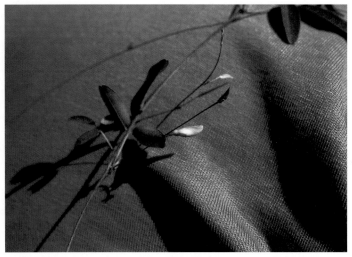

8. *Heles-here* "The good medicine," downy milk pea *Galactia volubilis* (L.) Britton

Heles-here is found in dry areas. Look for it around the base of a tree, because it is a vine that crawls on trees. It also crawls on high grass and can be in an open place as well. Search carefully because it is so small. Look for the top and follow the vine into the soil to get to the roots. Sometimes it is stored because it disappears in the winter. The leaves of the delicate vine are soft. I never saw flowers. The roots have little knots. Dig up the roots for the knots. Use the whole plant in medicine. Four of the vines with roots are usually used. The plant is used in medicines for babies and adults.

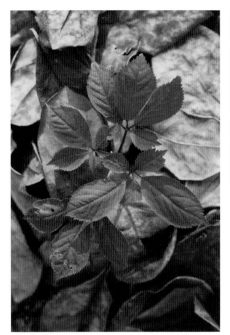

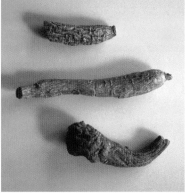

9. *Heles-hvtke* Ginseng *Panax quinquefolium* L.

The only place I have found white medicine is in Oklahoma in Norman's drugstore in Wewoka. Some health food stores have ginseng, but it is a different color than white and often not in the root form. I buy the roots, which sometimes are divided and long. *Heles-hvtke* is used for pain medicine and all kinds of other treatments, such as for shortness of breath and heart disease. It can be used dry or mixed in water. Just use a little bit. Sometimes just scrape it in the water. To treat the pain, doctors can put it in water, but sometimes they chew it and put the crushed ginseng directly on the place that hurts. Then wrap the area with white material.

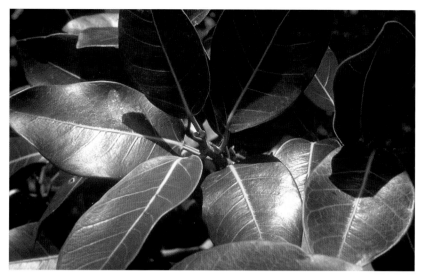

10. *Helokhakv*   Rubber plant, strangler fig   *Ficus aurea* Nutt.

This plant is found in the hammock, sometimes on a stump or wrapped around a cabbage tree (thus, strangler fig). The leaves are big and shiny and real green. Sometimes you can find a big plant, but mostly you find small ones. If you are going to use it for medicine, you have to collect four unopened leaves on the end of a branch. When you chop a branch, white milk comes out. Get it and put it in a can and boil it, and when it becomes gum, you chew it. In the past, we would get the milk on the brown leaves and put both in our mouths and chew it. If you chop the bark and let it melt down overnight, the next day you can get the gum off the tree and chew it. That's what we did when we were kids. My daddy told us he did that, too. (Slide by W. S. Judd.)

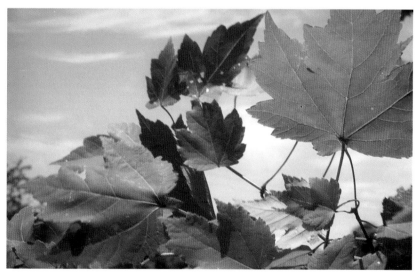

11. *Heno*   Red maple   *Acer rubrum* L.

You find this tree in a wet, swampy area, mostly around the roads. The leaves are white underneath and have three points. The stems are red. The seeds are red and grow in hanging clusters. The bark is used for women's treatment. Once in a while it is used for other medicine. For the women's treatment, you have to get a limb where it splits in two and get four pieces of the bark.

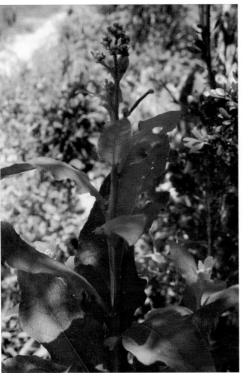

12. *Hetotvpe* Frost weed *Verbesina virginica* L.
Hetotvpe is used like *kvsvppē-heleswv,* for cold or cool medicine. If you get too hot while you are working over a fire, cold medicine is used to cool your body down. The plant has different-shaped leaves, some scalloped. It usually has one stem, which has green flanges down its sides. If you dig out the plant, it has a whole bunch of short worm-like roots. Usually four roots are used.

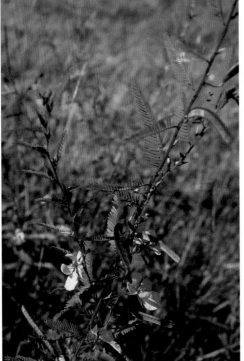

13. *Kowike entvlako* Quail's foot, partridge pea, or bird's foot trefoil *Chamaecrista fasciculata* Michx. Greene or *C. chamaecrista* L.
You can find this plant in an open place around a hammock in damp areas. The leaves are really small with a whole bunch on the stalk [a compound leaf]. It forms a bush with a yellow bloom. The seeds look like little beans. *Kowike entvlako* means "quail beans." This plant is sometimes called *svtv empvtakv.* When we were little, we would put *kowike entalakv* in a box and put *svtv* (custard apples) on it to ripen. We would check the box each day. When the *svtv* was orange or ripe, the stem would pull right out. We each got a *svtv* and were not allowed to share. I don't know why. If you eat *svtv* before it is ripe, people say that it will choke you. *Svtv* used to be prevalent in the area.

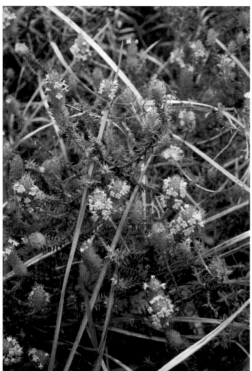

14. *Kvfockv*   Penny royal sage, peppermint
Pycnothymus rigidus Bart. or *Piloblephis
rigida*

Kvfockv is found in areas with pine trees on
dry land with palmettos around. It grows as
really green bushes. Its tiny leaves smell like
peppermint. My mother told us if you have
a cold you could smell this. It was good
smelling, so we would smell it all the time.
Kvfockv is used in different treatments. Usually one or two sprigs of the leaves are
needed.

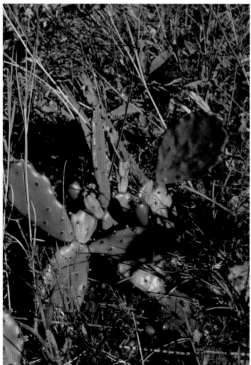

15. *Kvnrvkko*   Prickly pear   *Opuntia
humifusa* Raf.

Kvnrvkko is found on high, dry ground or
sometimes on flatland that is usually dry. It
has long spines and is green and flat, kind
of like a hog's ear but bigger. When it
breaks, it is wet, thick like glue but not
sticky. It has yellow flowers. Near the flowers it has fine little stickers. The fruit—what
we call the berries (*enlokcē*)—is red and
stands on the top of the flat paddlelike
parts. I heard that Spanish people eat the
fruit. It's good. I never used *kvnrvkko* for the
medicine until a man told me it was good
for sores. Get the roots, boil them, and put
them on the sores.

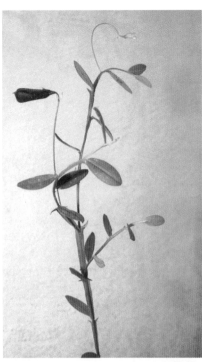

16. *Kvsvkakuce*   Rattle box, rabbit bells
Crotalaria pallida
You find this plant around the cabbage palms
and oak trees in an area that is not too wet.
One kind has round leaves, another has nar-
rower and longer leaves. The doctor tells you
what kind to get. Its seedpod looks like that
of a little pea; when it turns black and you
shake it, it rattles. *Kvsvkakuce* is used for
vwotickv, to throw up with, when using "on
the wagon" medicine. Collect four plants
with roots, stems, and leaves. Some people
use it for high blood pressure. For that treatment, four whole plants are collected, boiled,
and drunk; the medicine is used without the
Indian doctor's songs.

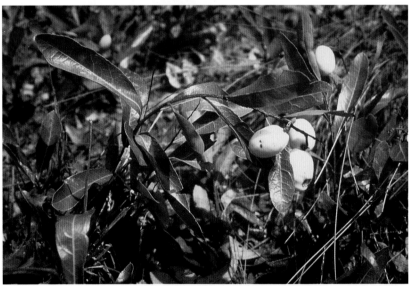

17. *Lucv-huehkv enhompetv*   Gopher turtle food, gopher apple   *Licania michauxii* Prance
Lucv-huehkv enhompetv is found in dry, sandy, hilly areas low to the ground. It only grows six
to eight inches high. The leaves are elongated with rounded ends. It has a little white flower
and a fruit that looks somewhat like a pecan but is a little bit bigger. The plant crawls along
the ground by an underground root system. It is named for the gopher turtle, which eats its
fruit. *Lucv-huehkv enhompetv* is used mostly in death medicine. When collecting, get the
whole plant, but the roots are especially important. (Slide by W. S. Judd.)

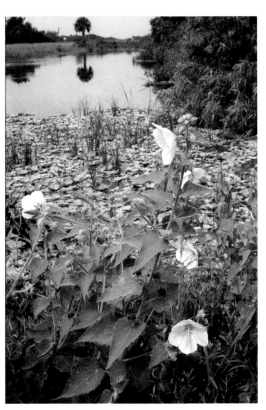

18. Opv 'mvhoswv or opv enhvfvtēhkv
Mallow *Malvacese*

A lot of *opv 'mvhoswv* grows along the road by the lake. The leaves look grayish. The flowers are pink and stand right by the stem. You collect the roots or whatever parts the doctor wants. I don't know what the plants are used for, but sometimes the doctor says, "Put some of those in the medicine."

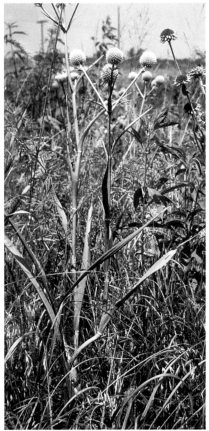

19. *Passv* Button snakeroot *Eryngium yucciafolium* Michx.

Look for *passv* in a dry open ground with palmettos around it. The leaves are long and slender and have little stickers on both sides. *Passv* blossoms arise on a little stem about two to three feet tall. The blooms are white. To collect the plant, dig it out of the ground to get the roots. Only one root is needed. Sometimes the medicine man asks for the root from a plant that does not have multiple roots, so you have to look carefully. When you look on top, the one with multiple roots will have a lot of heads. The single root will have just one head. The single one is hard to find. Prepare the root according to the doctor's instructions. The root can be used whole, cut in four pieces, or crushed. I think this is a strong medicine because it is the one used for the Green Corn Dance.

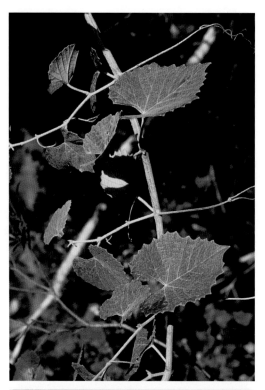

20. *Pvrko* Grape *Vitis rufotomentosa* or *Vitis shuttleworthii*

Pvrko grows the same way as *culoswuce*—on oak trees, on wax myrtles, and on fences. The vine has a brown stem with green leaves that are white and fuzzy underneath. *Pvrko* bears grapes, which are almost red and bigger than the fruit of *culoswuce*. *Pvrko* tastes sour; there is no sweet in it. Like *culoswuce*, it has tendrils for support. Watch out when you get this plant because it grows with poison ivy. In the wintertime, when the leaves of both plants have fallen, you can pick the wrong one easily. Collect four pieces with leaves and vines that are about four inches long. In the wintertime you can only get the vine. *Pvrko* is used for many kinds of medicine—whatever the doctor requires—like death medicine.

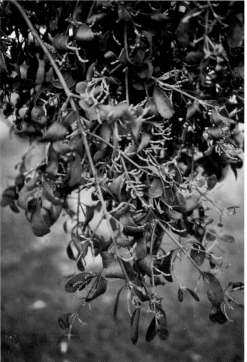

21. *Roheleko* Mistletoe *Phoradendron serotinum* Raf. M.C. Johnston or *P. flavescens* Pursh Nutt.

You can find *roheleko* in kind of wet areas with the Carolina ash trees. In other areas it is found easily in oak trees. The leaves are real green and rubbery. The plant grows on branches of the host tree. It looks like a ball on the limb. Since *roheleko* breaks very easily, it is not hard to pick once it is spotted, unless it is growing high in the tree. Then you have to climb the tree or use a stick to knock it down. If the tree is small enough, you can bend the branches to reach it. Get a small length of stem. You don't need a lot. (Slide by W. S. Judd.)

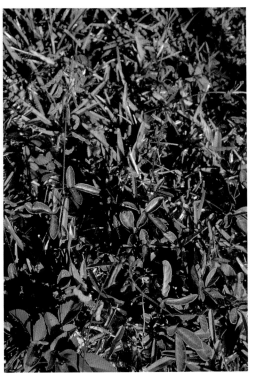

22. 'Stvlokpuce Beggar's lice *Desmodium lineatum* or *D. supinam*

'Stvlokpuce means "it sticks," like it sticks to your clothes. This little one that is found anywhere crawls on the ground and has thin leaves (about one inch) that are kind of soft and limber. Don't get the kind with the longer, stiff leaves. The flowers are yellow. The seeds look like little ol' beans strung together. Collect the beans and the stems with them, too. *'Stvlokpuce* is used for a lot of different things. It is used for alcoholic treatment, and someone told me that she used it for pregnant women near delivery.

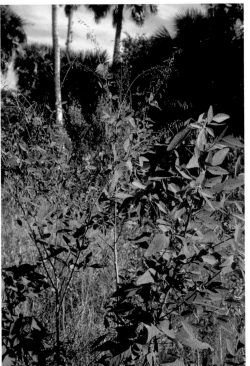

23. 'Stvlokpuce hvlwat Beggar's lice *Desmodium*

'Stvlokpuce hvlwat is like the other *'stvlokpuce* except that it is taller. The tall ones don't crawl on the ground, and the seeds stick straight up on top. *Hvlwat* means "tall" (singular); *hvlhvlwvt* refers to a bunch of tall ones growing together. *'Stvlokpuce hvlwat* is found around the road. In August, it has little beans that are ready to fall off. The plant looks like a little tree with little limbs. It grows in bunches (many plants together). The flower is yellow. Seeds are little half-ovals that stick to your clothes. Collect the seeds. I usually get a whole bunch and sometimes keep it on hand for times when it is not available. It is used for any kind of medicine but usually to make you throw up.

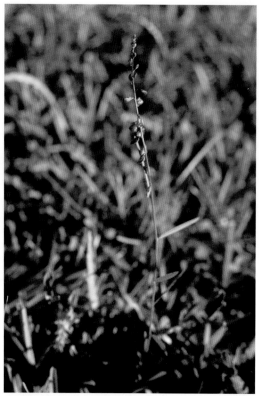

24. *Svpeyv* Small one, candy root, polygala *Polygala grandiflora* Walt.

You find this plant in an open place on dry or damp land. Get four whole plants with the roots attached. The thin stem is about a foot tall with small purple flowers, and the root is white. You use *svpeyv* for treatment to clean the body and to vomit. It is used in "on the wagon medicine" as well.

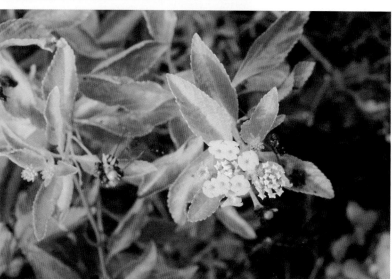

25. *Svpeyv rakko* Big one, lantana *Lantana camara* L.

This is the stronger of the *svpeyv* and called the "big one." It is found sometimes around the road and sometimes in a hammock in a dry or damp area. The leaves are kind of fuzzy, and the plant is bushy and low. The flowers bunch together and can be yellow, pink, or purple. Collect the roots or limbs for the medicine. *Svpeyv rakko* as used for the same things as the other *svpeyv*, but it is stronger.

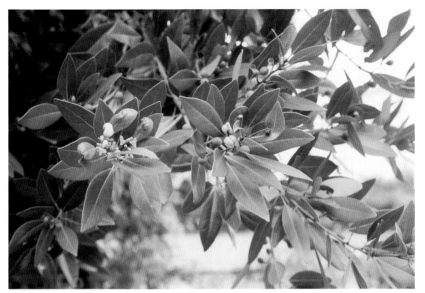

26. *Tolv*   Red bay   *Persea borbonia* L. Sprengel

Tolv grows like a tree and is frequently found growing inside a patch of palmetto or in an open flat land that is not too dry. When I find a tree, I remember where it is so I can find it easily next time. When I get *tolv* for healing, I go to a different tree than the one I used to collect death medicine. The shiny-looking leaves are long and stiff. Sometimes the tree has little black berries, but I have never seen blossoms on it. If you cut or crush the leaves, they smell strong. Some people use *tolv* for seasoning in foods like stews or spaghetti, but I have never used it in cooking nor have I known any Seminoles to use it in cooking. *Tolv* is used in most Indian treatments. It is usually the first thing you have to collect. It is used for protection and for healing. If the *tolv* will be used for death medicine, I pick branches from the west side of the plant. For healing, I use the east-side branches.

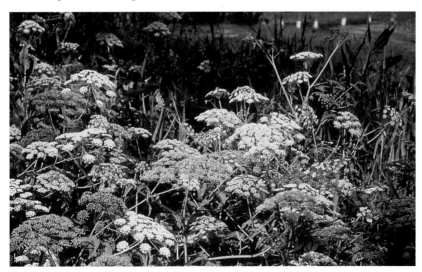

27. *Torkop-rakko*   Water hemlock   *Cicuta maculata* Coult. and Rose

Torkop-rakko is found in canals in or near the water. It has big green leaves, big stems, and white flowers. The stems have big joints. Get the roots and boil them. Put the liquid on the skin where the arthritis is. This medicine can also be used for itching. (Slide by W. S. Judd.)

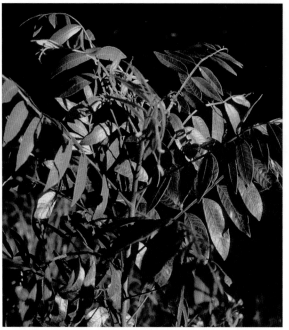

28. *Tvwv* Winged sumac *Rhus copallina* L.

Tvwv is found in palmetto patches, sometimes in open places. The leaf stem is about nine inches long, with oval-shaped leaves about two inches long on both sides of the stem. Sometimes the plants have flowers and berries. The berries are black when they are ripe, like elderberries, and grow in clusters. Collect the roots. To prepare them, wash, peel off the skin, and put them in water. Sometimes doctors use *tvwv* to make people on alcoholic treatment throw up or to make widows throw up to remove the breath of the deceased spouse.

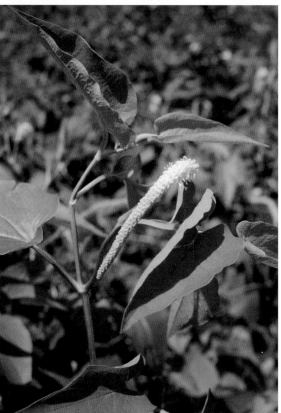

29. *Ue-heleswv* Lizard's tail *Saururus cernuus* L.

Ue-heleswv grows in water or in very wet ground around a creek, canal, or pond. Although not a vine, it looks similar to one. The leaves are heart shaped. The flower stalk looks like a little lizard's tail before the tiny white blossoms appear. The whole plant, but especially the white root, smells like peppermint. *Ue-heleswv* is used for all kinds of medicine. When you collect it, pull out the whole plant to get the roots. Both leaves and roots are used. Four plants are usually required.

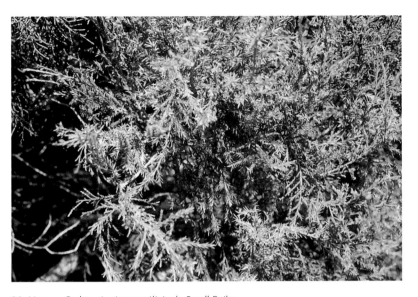

30. *Vcenv* Cedar *Juniperus silicicola* Small Bailey

Some people plant *vcenv* in their yards, so you can find it there once in a while. I get most of mine from Oklahoma, in kind of dry, rocky areas. There is some around on State Road 98 by Lake Okeechobee. *Vcenv* is a tree that has stickers. The seeds grow out of the top. Break off a limb to use in the medicine. You need just a little bit for the medicine, but if you get a limb you can save it for later. It is good to have on hand if a doctor calls for it. A lot of people burn it in the house, but I never did.

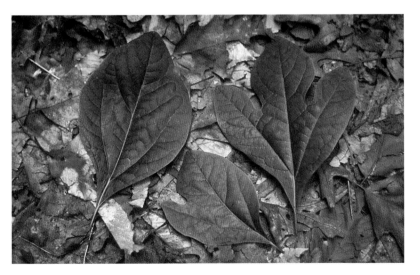

31. *Wēso* Sassafras *Sassafras albidum* Nutt. Nees

Wēso is a tree found in Oklahoma and in North Florida near Tallahassee. Look for it in a low area. In Oklahoma, ask permission to get onto the land to dig out the roots. Look for a young tree with a trunk about three inches in diameter. Dig it up to get the roots. Sometimes you need to pull out the tree with a truck. You can also buy *wēso* locally in a drugstore. *Wēso* is used for colds or a bad cough. Cut slivers of the bark off and boil them. Serve warm or hot like a tea. It is optional to have it treated by an Indian doctor. Four slivers of the bark can be included in other Indian medicines. Sometimes it is used to reduce blood sugar or for heart pain. (Slide by W. S. Judd.)

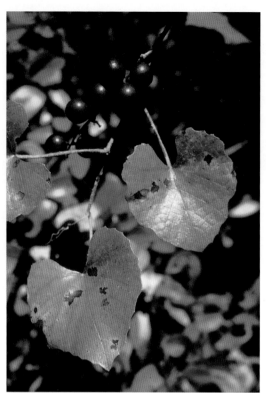

32. *Wotko empvrko*   Raccoon grapes   *Vitis cinerea*

The first time I found *Wotko empvrko* only on the Big Cypress Reservation, but now I find it not too far from the reservation on the south. It looks like wild grapes (*pvrko*), but it has leaves that are bigger and kind of fuzzy on the underside. Get the leaves and stem for medicine. If there are grapes on the vine, just leave them on. I have not used *Wotko empvrko* for a long time. It is used for owl sickness, which occurs when you are not able to sleep at night but sleep during the day. My mother told me not to eat the grapes of this plant.

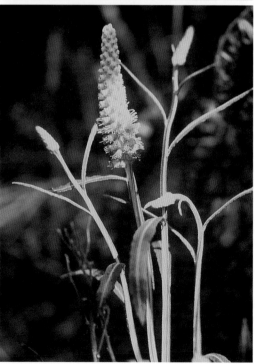

33. *Yvnvsv heleswv*   Black root   *Pterocaulon pycnostachyum*

Yvnvsv heleswv is found in dry, flat, sandy soil. Its name literally means "buffalo medicine." The leaves are green on top and whitish underneath. Overall, the plant has a gray cast with white flowers. The flower looks like a tail, with the blooms arising from the thick end, like a cattail. The stem has gray and green riblike projections, much like the stem of *hetotvpe*. Collect the roots, which grow in little knots. Usually four are used. (Slide by W. S. Judd.)

Treatment for Women after a Miscarriage to Prevent Another One

Hok·tv·ke en·he·les·ha·ye·tv es·tu·ce o·fvn e·le·pēt o·mat
(Yaa·too·che ha·yoo·ke en·we·shaa·kee·pa·ka e·ma·yek·cho·mee·ke)

Herbs to Collect

Creek name	Mikasuki name	English common name
1. *to·lv*	*too·le*	bay
2. *ak·wa·nv*	*o·ke·bak·she*	willow
3. *he·lok·ha·kv**	*ha·che·loo·paa·pe*	strangler fig or rubber tree
4. *e·to·hvt·kv***	*hee·kaa·pe*	Carolina ash
5. *he·no*	*a·shayk·ho·mee·che*	red maple
6. *cu·le*	*choo·ye*	slash pine
7. *yv·nv·sv he·les·wv****	*ya·na·she-ema·yek·che pe·chek·che a·lah·kah·che e·ma·yek·che*	black root

*Literally "gum making" for its white, sticky sap. This tree is in the ficus family and is generally found growing around a palmetto tree; hence the nickname, "strangler fig."
**Literally "white wood" for the appearance of the underside of branches. This tree is found in swampy areas in association with *ue·he·les·wv*.
***Literally "buffalo medicine."

The woman who gathers the medicine must not be having her period. The "Y" of the stems is needed for this treatment for all the herbs except *yvnvsv heleswv*. The Y is necessary because it looks like the split in a woman's legs. The inner sides of the Y of the stem are scraped out to put into the medicine. The root of the *yvnvsv heleswv* is used.

Take one red skirt and white thread to the doctor, maybe needles as well.

How to Use the Medicine

Mix the ingredients together in water and take them to the Indian doctor to be treated. (The doctor can be either male or female.) When using the medicine, heat it first. Use it on the body. Next boil it and steam the body with it. The patient may stand or sit over the steam. This treats the spirit inside the woman, which must be done before she becomes pregnant again.

After the medicine cools down, the woman may take a bath with it if she wants to. Use the medicine four days. At the end of four days, get a little bundle of *akwanv*, put it in water, and use it on the arms and legs but not the stomach. A little bit may be drunk at that time as well. The woman can now eat salt again.

Restrictions

· Do not eat anything with baking powder, anything that rises.
· Do not eat insides and backbones.
· No alcohol or tobacco.
· No salt.
· Do not lift heavy things.
· Do not sleep with a man for four months.
· Do not eat with others; eat alone, not with the group.
· Do not run.
· Do not step over logs.

This recipe was from Susie Billie and is used primarily for cleansing the woman. The medicine is used as well to heal a woman who's experienced ripping during childbirth.

Yvnvsv heleswv root is also used when girls have their first menstrual period. The girl has to be treated by a woman who is too old to have a period. By taking this medicine, the girl will not experience prolonged menstrual periods.

Treatment for Pregnant Women (to Protect the Baby)

Po·nvt·tv lvs·la·tat e·nok·ki·cv·ha·ne·kat e·mv·lek·ce·tv
(Nak-he·sah·ke los·loo·cha·ka e·no·kaa·chee·chah·te·ka e·ma·yek·cho·mee·ke)

Herbs to Collect

Creek name	Mikasuki name	English common name
He·les·he·re	*a·yek·che·hee·le*	downy milk pea

How to Use the Medicine

Get four plants of *heles-here* with the little balls on the roots. Mash up the balls and put it all in water. You can crush it with a hammer or wood. Take it to be treated with songs. Take a bath with it and drink four swallows. This makes the birth easier. After the woman takes a bath with it, the doctor has to fix it again if the doctor is nearby.

The woman takes this two or three weeks before she gives birth so the baby will be protected. Use the treatment like this for the baby after birth anytime before the baby is four months old to protect him or her. The baby will be pretty and healthy when born, and the birth will be easier.

Restrictions (until baby is four months old)

· Do not eat backbone.
· Do not eat deer.
· Do not eat turkey.

When a woman is pregnant there are a lot of restrictions. Women are prohibited from eating large amounts of food, or else the baby will be too big before it is born. The woman is not allowed to step over anything or to run.

Baby Treatments

He·les-he·re 'sak·lo·pē·ce·tv or
pos·sv·lē en·he·les-ha·ye·tv
(*A·yek·che-hee·le sho·bah·lee·chee·ke* or *po·sa·leh·che e·ma·yek·cho·mee·ke*)

After a baby is born, the father gets *tolv* and *akwanv*. He puts them in a big pot and mixes them with water. He takes them to the Indian doctor to be fixed. Next, he invites the community people who want to use this medicine. They can use it there or take it home with them. Keep the rest of the medicine to use for two or three days. There are no restrictions.

Tolv is the number one Indian medicine used. Before a woman goes to the hospital to have a baby or before one is born at home, *tolv* is rubbed all over the woman's body. It keeps evil spirits away.

When a woman and her baby come home from the hospital, they will crush up *tolv* and put it on their bodies in the car.

A bundle is made of *tolv* to put on a baby when it is born. *Tolv* is placed in the house or burned in the house to keep the child from having bad dreams. It can be used for others who have bad dreams.

When hanging or burning *tolv*, you do not need to have it treated, but the bundles that the baby wears need to be treated first.

Treatment for When the Baby Won't Eat

Take white grits (*osafke hvtke*) to the doctor to be treated. Cook the grits and feed the baby four spoonfuls, then let the baby eat the rest.

Treatment for Babies Who Cry in the Evening All the Time

Go see a doctor and explain what is happening. The doctor will ask for *tolv* and then treat it. Crush the *tolv* and rub the baby with it. Burn the *tolv* for the baby to smell or hold it close to the baby. Then put a bundle of *tolv* on the baby or put a bundle of it with him or her for four days.

How to Make a Bundle of *Tolv* for a Baby

A little *tolv* is saved from the leaves that are treated to take to the hospital. It is kept near the baby until he or she is four months old. The dried leaves are crushed. You make a tiny bag of heavy material, so it won't come apart if the baby chews it. You fill it with *tolv* and tie it real tight. It is pinned on the baby's shirt or tied on the string of white beads around the neck. Instead of *tolv*, we used to save the hair from the baby's first haircut at four months. The cut hair was then placed in a little bundle and tied to the baby's necklace.

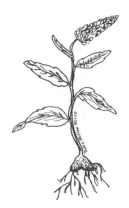

Treatment for Milk for Baby Bottles to Keep Baby from Throwing Up

Take baby's milk (*wa·kv pe·sē*) to the Indian doctor to be treated. Then give the treated bottle of milk to the baby to drink. Give the doctor money or four yards of yellow material.

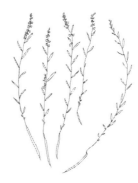

Treatment to Protect the Baby from His Father's Touch

Es·tu·ce pos·sv·lē·ho·cat en·he·les·ha·ye·tv
(*Yaa·too·che po·sa·leh·che e·ma·yek·cho·mee·ke*)

Herbs to Collect

Creek name	Mikasuki name	English common name
1. *to·lv*	*too·le*	bay
2. *he·les·he·re*	(*a·yek·che·hee·le*)	downy milk pea

If the father has been with a woman other than the mother, the baby will get sick if the father touches the other woman and then touches the baby. Medicine is used to protect the baby.

How to Use the Medicine

Use four whole plants of *heles-here:* stem, root, and leaves. Crush the roots of *heles-here* and put them in water with the other parts and *tolv.* Get the medicine treated by a doctor. Give the baby a little drink four times. Bathe the baby with it. When the medicine gets low, add water and return it to the doctor to be treated. Do this four times. Then give white grits to the doctor and let him fix it. Give the baby four spoons of the grits. After the four spoons, feed the rest to the baby.

Restrictions for the mother (four months)

If the mother is nursing, she cannot eat the following:
• soft stuff;
• soft-shell turtle;
• catfish;
• internal organs;
• backbones.
If the baby is using a bottle, there are no restrictions.

Use the same medicine for babies and toddlers when they don't want to eat or they get mad all the time.

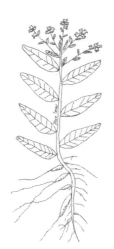

Treatment to Be "On the Wagon"

V·wo·tic·kv
(Sha·woo·taa·chee·ke)

Treatment One: Herbs to Collect

Creek name	Mikasuki name	English common name
1. *to·lv*	*too·le*	bay
2. *sv·pe·yv*	*a·woo·taa·chee·ke em a·yek·che*	Polygala
or substitute *sv·pe·yv rak·ko*	*sha·pe·ye choo·be*	lantana
3. *kv·sv·ka·ku·ce*	*sha·cha·chap·koo·che*	rattlebox, rabbit bells
4. *cv·to os·tet*	*ta·le shee·taa·ken*	four smooth stones
5. *ak·wa·nv* (optional)	*o·ke·bak·she*	willow
6. *sv·pe·yv·lo·poc·ku·ce* (optional)	*sha·pe·ye·pes·kosh·ka*	candy root

When you collect *svpeyv,* gather the whole plant, including roots. If you use *svpeyv rakko,* use the leaves and blossoms. *Svpeyv rakko* is stronger and has different requirements.

When being treated, take two or four yards of yellow material for the Indian doctor. If *svpeyv rakko* is used, the doctor requires a live hog as well.

Treatment Two: Herbs to Collect

Creek name	Mikasuki name	English common name
1. *to·lv*	*too·le*	bay
2. *kv·sv·ka·ku·ce*	*sha·cha·chap·koo·che*	rattlebox, rabbit bells
3. *cv·to os·tet*	*ta·le shee·taa·ken*	four smooth stones

Take four yards of yellow and four yards of red material for the treatment. The two treatments are the same except for the use of *svpeyv* and the items they require. Both of these treatments are the strongest treatments because they have a stone in them. If the doctor doesn't use a stone, the treatment is not strong, but the restrictions are the same.

If you want to use "on the wagon" medicine or just "wagon" medicine, go to an Indian doctor and tell him what you want. He will ask if you will obey the restrictions for four months. He will say, "I do not like to see my treatment broken." He will say, "Get medicine *tolv, svpeyv,* and *kvsvkakuce* and *cvto ostet.*" When you get it all together, put it in water and take it back to the doctor. Let him fix it for you and give it back to you. He will tell you how to use it.

How to Use the Medicine

Dig a hole to vomit in. In the morning before you eat, take the medicine to the hole. Drink the medicine until you get full and vomit with it four times the first morning. If the medicine gets low, add more water. Do this four times the same morning. After you finish, cover the hole with leaves, not dirt. Do not eat or go back to sleep until noon or stay in the house all day.

When using *vwotickv,* you need some willow you got fixed at the same time you got the medicine. If you use the willow, you can eat anything you want and get out of the house, but obey the other restrictions for four months. You are not to break restrictions like cigarettes. You can wait four days after you take the medicine. If you need the cigarettes badly, you can take them back to the same doctor to be treated for use.

Restrictions

· No alcohol, beer, or wine for four months.
· No cigarettes or other tobacco.
· No backbones.
· No animal organs or insides (chitlins, liver, etc.).
· No combing hair for two to four days.
· No going out; stay inside and don't look around too far for two to four days.

Restrictions (when using *svpeyv rakko*)

· Stay in the house for one day.
· Do not watch television for one day.
If the restrictions are broken, the condition will worsen.

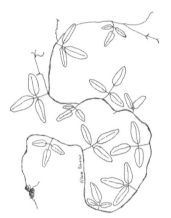

Death Medicine

To·lv tak·hue·rv
(Yaa·te e·lee·pan om·me·ka e·ma·yek·che)

Herbs to Collect

Creek name	Mikasuki name	English common name
1. *to·lv*	*too·le*	bay
2. *ak·wa·nv*	*o·ke·bak·she*	willow
3. *pvr·ko*	*baɬ·be*	wild grapes
4. *cu·los·wu·ce*	*cho·koo·che*	little muscadine grapes, wild raisins
5. *kv·foc·kv*	*ha·po·she·kaa·ye·choo·be*	penny royal sage, peppermint
6. *ca·fvk·nv*	*o·la·ke*	huckleberry
7. *lu·cv·hueh·kv en·hom·pe·tv*	*a·paa·ho·she em·em·pee·ke*	gopher turtle food
8. *ro·he·le·ko*	*hen·ɬe 'mas·hok·che*	mistletoe
9. *ue·he·les·wv*	*yah·ka·ka·yek·che*	lizard's tail

Collect all ingredients. Leaves gathered from trees or scrubs like *tolv*, *pvrko*, and *culoswuce* should be selected from the east side of the plant. A lot of *tolv* is needed for death medicine, some for the medicine and some for burning. I used to get two bunches for the medicine, but now the doctors ask for three. One or two bunches are used for the medicine pot, and one is used for burning. Just the leaves are used for the medicine pot, but both stem and leaves are burned. Strip four pieces of bark from *akwanv* to use. The more bark, the redder and stronger the mixture. Roots are gathered from *lucv-huehkv enhompetv* and *ue-heleswv*. Break the herbs into smaller pieces and place them in a paper bag. Take them to the Indian doctor to be treated. The treated *tolv* is used dry by the kinfolk. They chew a little and rub some on their bodies before they view or touch the deceased's body, remove what belongs to the dead person, or before they go to sleep.

When you take it to the doctor, he or she may ask you for four yards each of black, red, white, and yellow material; a deer skin with the head on; an ax; a knife; and one hog. On the fourth day, give the doctor a gun if the family uses a gun.

Restrictions (four months or until the new moon)

· No catfish, garfish, or mudfish.
· No chicken or turkey.
· No liver or chitlins.
· No hog's head cheese, pork chops, or pig's feet.
· No beer or wine (or other alcohol) and no cigarettes.
· No soft-shell turtle.
· No pumpkin.
· No fawn.
· No backbones.

If the person wants to eat chicken, he or she can cut off a little piece and put it in the medicine. Then it is all right to eat.

How to Use the Medicine

After the person is buried, put ingredients in large pot and cover them with water. Set the pot beside the fire on the west side and heat the contents. Drink four swallows of the medicine after you come back from the burial and put it on your body. Let it sit there for four days. In the past, the medicine was used four times; now it is sometimes used just one day, depending upon the family.

After the medicine pot is finished (after four days), the Indian doctor keeps the medicine pot. Then everyone is supposed to clean up the yard, cooking pots, and everything else. After that, all the people have to go out to take a bath in a canal or wherever they find water. After they use the soap, the rest of the soap must be thrown in the water. When they return to the house, they get lard or grease, and everyone puts it on their bodies.

When they are ready to eat, they have to cook *osafke* in the medicine fire after it has been cleaned and before they eat the rest of the food. After four days, when they are going to eat fresh meat, they have to put it on the fire a little while before they boil it. The meat does not have to be put on the fire if it is fried.

In the old days, the dead person's possessions went to his or her family of origin. Now they are given to the deceased's children.

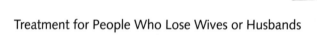

Treatment for People Who Lose Wives or Husbands

Em·pvl·se som·kē·pat en·he·les·ha·ye·tv
(Shen·tok·lee·ke en·wes·haa·kee·pa·ka e·ma·yek·cho·mee·ke)

Herbs to Collect

Creek name	Mikasuki name	English common name
1. *to·lv*	*too·le*	bay
2. *pas·sv*	*pa·she*	button snakeroot
3. *tv·wv*	*he·ko·taa·pe*	bitter wood, winged sumac

Gather the roots of the *passv* and *tvwv*. Use one root from *passv* and cut it into four pieces. Collect many roots of the *tvwv*, specifically the bark of the roots of one tree, which makes a person throw up. The herbs are mixed with water in a gallon jar.

How to Use the Medicine

You have to take this treatment after four days following the death and before four months have passed. After that, you ask a collector to get the

Indian medicine so you can throw up, to clean your insides. Treatment keeps you from being too lonely. The medicine and some *osafke hvtke* (white grits) are treated by an Indian doctor. Drink the medicine before breakfast until you are full and throw up. Do this four times. Sit down in front of the doctor, who then pours the medicine on your head and gives you a bath. You take a bath with the treated solution for four days in the morning, and you are given *osafke hvtke*.

Someone who has already lost a spouse is the only one who can take care of you. That person already went through the process and knows what to do. It is okay to give the treatment even after remarrying. A lot of people won't do it because they don't have any faith in it and they are scared. Others are afraid to do that if their spouse is alive.

A woman's kinfolk are the ones who are going to do it for the first time. First the kin takes you to the water—a canal or pond—and asks you to go under water four times. You have to eat food by yourself and without salt for four days. You're the only one who will drink *osafke* with just grits and water cooked together. The *osafke* is put in a little pot where you drink by yourself and coffee, too.

Restrictions

You eat alone for four months even at a restaurant. If you're a man and do not want to cook, widows can come and cook for you. You are not to eat anything with baking powder (anything that rises). Crackers are okay. You can use plain flour to make bread, but no baking powder. In addition:
· No pork.
· No turkey.
· No better catfish.
· No soft-shell turtle.
· No mudfish.
· No little deer or fawn.
· No garfish.
· No backbones.
· No insides.

Before four months, you have to throw up with the medicine. After four months, you have to see the new moon before the last treatment is given. The kin who has lost a spouse has to take you to the water. You wear new clothes. You throw away all the old clothes you were wearing when your mate was alive. When my husband died, I had to gather all the clothes that I wore with him. If other widows can get the good clothes, they can have them. I got new clothes after four months and threw away all the clothes I wore for the four months. Everything is finished after four months.

When the Green Corn Dance comes, if you want to go, the one working with you will take you to the Green Corn Dance to watch the ball game. Next, you watch the last four dances, and that is it. As the people dance, your helper gives you a swallow of whiskey four times. After that you cut it off, but it is up to you whether to have any more. Whiskey is the finishing part of the medicine. It is up to you to join in and dance all night or go home.

6

Remedies

♦♦♦♦♦♦♦♦♦♦♦♦♦♦♦♦♦

ak·tv·pē·hv-rak·ko	A water plant with heart-shaped leaves. Leaves contain a padding of air, which keeps them afloat. For sores, use a piece of the root.
a·tak·rv lvs·te	For kidney problems.
ca·fak·nv (huckleberry)	Good for anything.
'co·he·ce·ko (blind deer plant)	Ingredient for cough medicine.
'co·mv·hv (deer potato)	For knots in stomach.
cu·fe 'mvs·sv (rabbit medicine)	For muscle cramps; use in hot water as a tea or heat and breathe the steam.
cu·le (pine)	For sores: crush and boil tender new growth.
cu·le e·moh·lo·wa·ku·ce (white bud on pine)	To clean sores: boil and add *tolv*.
e·co em·pv·ka·nv (hog's plum)	For arthritis.
e·co hvc·ko v·ha·kv (deer ears)	For arthritis of bones: use whole plant.
e·fv·kv-la·nu·ce (yellow vine)	For arthritis: mix with alcohol, and apply it when it turns black. Learned from Oklahoma people.
en·kv·to·po·kv lvs·te (sunflower, black-eyed Susan)	For pain and swelling in the breast. Dig up all of the plant and boil it. Apply to areas as a warm wash or heat just the plant.
es·pas·kv·ha·kv	For kidney problems. The name's literal translation is "like a broom." Boil the root, then drink it. It makes you pass water. This information came from an Oklahoma doctor.
ha·lo·sv·ka·tv en·ti·hv (moccasin vine or climbing hemp weed)	For snake bites.

93

he·lv·pv en·he·les·wv	For ringworm.
(sundew)	
he·to·tv·pe	Cold medicine.
(frost weed)	
ko·wi·ke en·tv·la·ko	For high blood pressure. If you find a single
(quail bean)	stem, get the roots and boil them to make a tea to
	drink to pass water. From Oklahoma.
kv·foc·kv	For congestion: boil and breathe the steam.
(peppermint)	
o·pv 'mv·hos·wv	For cramps, heat and put on area.
(owl threads)	
o·pv en·hv·fv·tēh·kv	Will force labor.
(owl boots)	
po·yv·fek·cv e·kv·hes·se cvp·ko	For depression.
(long ghost hair)	
pv·he hvt·ke,	For headache.
pv·he hvt·ku·ce	
(white grass)	
pv·to ca·tu·ce	For ringworm.
(red fungus)	
sak·co·me·to	For alligator sickness (when an alligator makes
(button bush)	you sick).
'stv·lok·pu·ce	Used when you don't feel like eating and throw
(beggar's lice)	up (called the "snake sickness" or "dream about
	snakes").
tar·tah·kv	For aching bones and broken bones: boil the
(white ash from Oklahoma)	bark, and wash with it four times in the morning
	and for four days.
to·lv	A main ingredient in medicines.
(bay)	
tor·kop-rak·ko	For arthritis pain or itch. Boil the plant
(water hemlock)	and apply it to the area.
ue-he·les·wv	An ingredient in treatments after a death.
(lizard's tail)	
v·ce·nv	Burn the plant in the house to keep bad spirits
(cedar)	away. In the past it was used in death medicine.
wē·so	For cough or diarrhea. Usually imported from
(sassafras)	Oklahoma but may be found in northern Florida;
	use the bark to make tea.
ya·mē·li·kv	For swelling, peel off the bark of the root and put
	it in hot water. Apply warm to the swollen area.
yv·nv·sv he·les·wv	To stop heavy menstrual flow, boil the root and
(buffalo medicine)	drink the tea.

7

Plant Identification Chart
for Creek Speakers

◆◆◆◆◆◆◆◆◆◆◆◆◆◆◆◆◆◆◆

Creek name	Mikasuki name	English name[1]	Botanical name
ahatkv	ahe-halbe	white ash	*Populus*
akkotorkv	—	lotus	*Nelumbo lutea*
aktvpēhv	akpolohlooche	floating hearts, water floater	*Nymphoides aquaticum* Walt. Kunte
akwanv	okebakshe	willow	*Salix amphibia*[2]
asvn-hvtkuce	ashoome-hatkooche	British soldiers	—
cafaknv	olake	huckleberry, Darrow blueberry	*Vaccinium darrovii* Camp.
catv-folotv	—	beauty berry	*Callicarpa americana* L.
cetto enheleswv	chente ayekche	*snake medicine, clematis*	*Clematis baldwinii* Torri & Gray
'coheceko	eeche chaatehche	*blind deer plant, goldenrod*	*Solidago fistulosa* P. Miller or *S. canadensis* L.
'compvkanv	eeche entohaane	*deer peaches*	*Ximenia americana* L.
'comvhv	eeche 'mahe	*deer potato*	*Liatris laxa*
coskelpv	taapooche	elderberry	*Sambucus simpsoni*
cufe 'mvssv	chokfe empataake	*rabbit's bed, panic grass*	*Panicum zalapense* H.B.K. or *P. polycaulon* Nash
cule	chooye	slash pine	*Pinus caribaea* Morelet
cule emohlowakuce	chooye enlepaatooche, chooye ebeele	pine tip	*Pinus caribaea* Morelet
culoswuce	chokooche	*wild raisins, little muscadine grape, scuppernong, little fox grape*	*Cissus munsoniana* Simpson
cvto ostet	tale sheetaaken	*four smooth stones*	—
eco empvkanv	eeche entohaane	deer peaches, hog's plum	*Ximenia americana* L.
eco hvcko vhakv	eeche hakchobe	deer ears, sun-bonnet	*Chaptalia tomentosa* Vent.
eco nokwvnayv	—	—	*Cynanchum*
efvkv-lanuce	fayte ememrepeeke[3]	*golden threads, love vine*	*Cassytha filiformis* Lauraceae
ēkvnv cokhesse	yakne chooshke	*ground whiskers*	*Rhynchospora divergens* Chapm. Ex M.A. Curtis[4]

enkvtopokv-lvste	emalopeeke looche	black-eyed Susan	*Rudbeckia hirta* L.
espaskvhakv	—	*broom plant*	*Euthamia minor* Michx. Greene
este hvlwat cokhesse	yaat-chayhe echooshke	*tall person's whiskers*	*Tillandsia setacea* SW or *Vitarria lineata* L.
este lopockuce or este-lopocke emeto	yaat-hoboske emahe	*where the little people live*	bundles of needles of *Pinus caribaea* Morelet
este-sumkat entvpentv	ewaashaake entapente	fern that grows in a cabbage palm	—
eto-hvtkv, 'to-hvtkv	heekaape	Carolina ash	*Fraxinus caroliniana* Miller
halosvkatv entihv	wahole entayhe	moccasin vine, climbing hemp weed	*Mikania scandens* L. Willdenow
hefepe or hefepe-nërkv	hefepe-eele	bottle gourd seeds	*Lagenaria sicearia* Mol.
heles-here	ayekche-heele	*good medicine,* downy milk pea	*Galactia volubilis* L. Britton
heles-hvtke	ayekche-hatke	ginseng	*Panax quinquefolium* L.
helokhakv	hache loopaape	strangler fig, rubber tree	*Ficus aurea* Nutt.
helvpv enheleswv	—	sundew	*Drosera rotundifolia* L.
heno	ashayk-fomeeche	red maple	*Acer rubrum* L.
hesse-tvpehv	heshke takhe	wide leaf	*Brassica oleracea* L.
hetotvpe	eptaape	ice plant, frost weed	*Verbesina virginica* L.
hoktvlkolowv enlocowv vhakuce	kolotpahche ayekche	*old lady's paint pot, wide-open sore medicine,* hog food	*Ludwigia virgata* Michx.
hvlpvtv etolaswv vhakv	halpate choklaashe	gator tongue, blue iris	*Crinum americanum* L.[5]
kowike entvlako	kowaashe empataake	quail bean, partridge pea, or bird's foot trefoil	*Chamaecrista fasciculata* Michx. or *C. chamaecrista* L.
kvco	—	green briar	*Smilacaceae auriculata*
kvfockv	haposhekaaye-choobe	peppermint, penny royal sage	*Pycnothymus rigidus* Bart.
kvnrvkko	—	prickly pear	*Opuntia humifusa* Raf.
kvsvkakuce	shachachapkooche	rattle box, rabbit bells	*Crotalaria pallida* or *C. rotundifolia* Walt. Gmel.
lakcv-cvmpv sohhontat	okecheske entapente	resurrection fern	*Polypodium polypodioides* L. Watt.

Creek name	Mikasuki name	English name[1]	Botanical name
lakcv-cvmpv tafvmpuce vhakusat sohhontusat	yooshnokaacheehche emayekche	wild orchid	—
lakcv-cvmpv vloklopusat	hamoohche loope entapente okecheske empakte	lichen	—
lucv-huehkv enhompetv	apaahoshe emempeeke 'stapoochkeeke	*gopher turtle food*, gopher apple	*Licania michauxii* Prance
meskolvpe		live oak	*Quercus virginiana*
opv enhvfvtēhkv	oopaake oshtaape shapoke	*owl boots*, mallow	Malvacese
opv 'mvhoswv	oopaake embakshe	*owl threads*, mallow	Malvacese
orko-latkv	olke	flag pawpaw[6]	—
passv	pashe	button snakeroot	*Eryngium yucciafolium* Michx.
poyvfekcv ekvhesse fvske	sholoopaale entokafaske	*sharp hair spirits*	—
poyvfekcv ensukcv-tvpekse	sholoopaale enshokpachakfe	ghost bug or insect chrysalis	—
pvhe hvtke or pvhe hvtkuce	pahe hatkooche	*small white grass* / sedge	*Pityopsis* sp.[7]
pvrko	balbe	grape	*Vitis rufotomentosa* or *V. shuttleworthii* House
pvto catuce	pakte keteschooche, shokhe-hatke hakchobe	red fungus	—
roheleko	henle 'mashokche	mistletoe	*Phoradendron serotinum* (Raf.) M.C. Johnston or *P. flavescens* (Pursh) Nutt.[8]
sakcometo	halpate-mashoshoote	*alligator shader*, common button bush	*Cephalanthus occidentalis* L.
'stvlokpuce	tofoome	beggar's lice	*Desmodium lineatum* or *D. supinam*
sulecvpe	showaane 'mochaape	wax myrtle	*Myrica cerifera* L.
svpeyv	wootaacheeke em oekekche	polygala	*Polygala grandiflora* Walt., *P. lutea*, or *P. regelii*
svpeyv hvlwat	tofoome-chayhe	—	—
svpeyv-lopockuce	shapeye-peshkooshka	candy root	—

Creek	Mikasuki	English	Scientific name
svpeyv rakko	shapeye-choobe	lantana	*Lantana camara* L.
tartahkv	—	white ash or cottonwood	*Populus*
tohome	ayekche-hoome	bitterwood	—
'to-hvtkv, eto-hvtkv	heekaape	Carolina ash	*Fraxinus caroliniana* Miller
tolv	toole	red bay	*Persea borbonia* L. Sprengel
torkop-rakko	etolpe-choobe	big joint plant, water hemlock	*Cicuta maculata* L.[9]
totkv cokhesse	yakne chooshke	*fire whiskers*	*Octoblepahrum albidum* Hedv.
tvkrv-lvste	atakle looche	little dog fennel	*Eupatorium capillifolium* Lam. Small
tvwv	hekotaape	winged sumac	*Rhus copallina* L.
ue-heleswv	yahkaka-yekche	lizard's tail	*Saururus cernuus* L.
vcenv	achene	cedar	*Juniperus silicicola* Small Bailey
vktvpēhv	akpolohlooche	*water floater, floating hearts*	*Nymphoides aquaticum* (Walt.) Kunte
vtakrv	atakle	dog fennel	*Eupatorium capillifolium* Lam. Small
welanv	laykaape	*stink plant, wormseed*	*Chenopodium ambrosiodes* L.
wēso	chahkane	sassafras	*Sassafras albidum* Nutt. Nees
wotko elupe	shaawe loope	raccoon or coon liver	*Stenandrium floridanum*
wotko empvrko	shaawe embalbe	raccoon grapes	*Vitis cinerea*
yamēlikv	ayekche-choobe	*wolf's food*	*Chrysobalanus oblongifolius* Michx.
yvnvsv heleswv	pechekche emayekche	buffalo medicine, black root	*Pterocaulon pycnostachyum* Michx. Ellis

Appendixes

Appendix A. List of Herbs in Alice's Repertoire

(with her phonetic pronunciation guide)

◆◆◆◆◆◆◆◆◆◆◆◆◆◆◆◆◆◆◆

English names in italics are literal translations. Italics under Creek and Mikasuki names are Alice's phonetic guide.

Creek name	Mikasuki name	English common name
1. akhatkv *uck·haht·kuh*	ahe-halbe *uh·he·hull·bee*	—
2. akwanv *uk·wa·nuh*	okebakshe *o·ke·buc·se*	willow
3. asvn-hvtkuce *ah·sun hut·ko·che*	ashoome-hatkooche *ah·shoe·me hot·koo·che*	British soldiers
4. atvkrv-lvste *ah·duk·thuh luhs·te*	atakle looche *ah·tak·de lo·che*	dog fennel
5. cafaknv *cha·fak·na*	olake *o·lak·ee*	huckleberry
6. catv-folotv *chah·duh fo·lo·duh*	—	beauty berry
7. cetto enheleswv *cheet·do in·he·lis·wuh*	chente ayekche *chen·de ah·yeek·che*	*snake medicine*, clematis
8. 'coheceko *co·hee·che·ko*	eeche chaatehche *ee·che cha·tee·che*	*blind deer plant*
9. culoswuce *ja·los·wa·ge*	chokooche *cho·koo·che*	wild raisins
10. 'compvkanv *e·chum·ba·kon·na*	eeche entohaane *e·ge en·toe·haht·ne*	*deer peaches*
11. 'comvhv *chu·ma·ha*	eeche 'mahe *e·che·mah·he*	*deer potato*
12. coskelpv *chos·kil·pv*	taapooche *dah·poo·che*	elderberry

13. cufe 'mvssv
chew·fe muh·suh
chokfe empataake
choke·fe em·bah·tah·ke
rabbit medicine, panic grass

14. cule emohlowakuce
chew·le en·moe·lo·vah·koo·che
chooye enlepaatooche, chooye ebeele
choo·ye en·le·pah·too·che, choo·ye e·beeth·le
pine tip

15. cvto ostet
chuh·do o·stet
tale sheetaaken
ta·le she·tah·ken
four smooth stones

16. eco hvcko vhakv
e·cho hutch·ko un·hah·guh
eeche hakchobe
e·che hak·cho·be
deer ears

17. efvkv-lanuce
e·fuh·kuh lah·nu·che
fayte emempeeke
fay·te e·mem·pee·ke
golden threads, love vine

18. ākvnv cokhesse
e·kuh·nuh choke·his·se
yakne chooshke
yak·ne choosh·ke
ground whiskers

19. enkvtopokv-lvste
en·kuh·bo·poh·kuh luhs·te
emalopeeke looche
e·ma·lo·pee·ke loo·che
black-eyed Susan

20. espaskvhakv
es·bas·kah·hah·kuh
—
broom plant

21. este hvlwat cokhesse
is·tee hul·what e·kuh his·se uh·hah·ku·che
yaat-chayhe echooshke
yaht·chay·he e·choos·ke
tall person's whiskers

22. este lopockuce or este-lopocke emeto
is·de lo·boch·ke or is·de lo·boch·ke e·me·do
yaat-hoboske emahe
yaht·ho·bos·ke e·mah·he
where the little people live

23. este-sumkat entvpentv
is·tee some·kuh en·tuh·ben·tuh
ewaashaake entapente
e·wah·shaw·ke en·da·ben·te
fern that grows in a cabbage palm

24. halosvkatv entihv
hah·lo·suh·ka·duh en·tay·huh
wahole entayhe
vvuh·ho·the en·tay·hee
moccasin vine, climbing hemp weed

25. hefepe or hefepe-nērkv
he·fe·be neethl·kuh
hefepe-eele
he·fe·be eeth·le
bottle gourd seeds

Creek name	Mikasuki name	English common name
26. heles-here *he·lis heeth·lee*	ayekche-heele *ah·yeek·che heeth·le*	*good medicine, downy milk pea*
27. heles-hvtke *he·lis hut·ke*	ayekche-hatke *ah·yeek·chee-hut·ke*	ginseng root
28. helokhakv *he·loke·hah·kuh*	hache loopaape *hah·che loo·bah·be*	rubber tree, strangler fig
29. heno *he·no*	ashayk-fomeeche *ah·shake fomeech·he*	red maple
30. hesse-tvpēhv *his·see duh·be·huh*	heshke takhe *hish·ke tak·he*	*wide leaf*
31. hetotvpe *he·toe·da·be*	eptaape *ep·ta·be*	*ice trée*
32. hoktvlkolowv enlocowv vhakuce *hok·dul·ko·low·wuh en·lo·cho·wuh uh·ha·ku·che*	kolotpahche ayekche *go·lot·pah·che a·yeek·che*	*old lady's paint pot, hog food*
33. hvlpvtv etolaswv vhakv *hul·put·tuh e·toe·las·wuh uh·hah·kuh*	halpate choklaashe *hal·pah·te choke·lah·she*	*gator tongue*, blue iris
34. hvtke-kafkv *hut·ke kaf·fuh*	waacheeshtafanke *wah·cheesh·tah·fun·ke*	cow food
35. kowike entvlako *ko·way·ke en·tah·lah·ko*	kowaashe empataake *ko·wah·she em·pah·dah·ke*	quail beans, partridge pea, bird's foot trefoil
36. kvfockv *kuh·foch·ka*	hapooshe kaaye-choobe *ha·pu·she ka·ye·cho·bee*	*peppermint*, penny royal sage
37. kvsvkakuce *ka·sa·ka·ko·che*	shachachapkooche *sa·cha·chup·ko·che*	rattle box, rabbit bells

38. lakcv-cvmpv sohhontat *lock·chuh chum·puh so·hon·tat*	okecheske entapente *o·ke·ches·ke en·da·ben·te*	resurrection fern
39. lakcv-cvmpv tafvmpuce vhakusat sohhontusat *lock·chuh-chum·buh dah·fum·poo·che* *uh·hah·ku·sot so·hon·doe·sot*	yooshnokaacheehche emayekche *yoosh·no·kah·chee·che e·mah·yeek·che*	wild orchid
40. lakcv-cvmpv vloklopusat *luck·chuh-chum·buh uh·loke·lowu·bo·zat*	hamoohche loope entapente okecheske empakte *huh·moe·chee lowu·bee in·tuh·pin·tee* *o·kee·chee·ski em·bak·tee*	lichen
41. lucv-huehkv enhompetv *lu·cha·we·ka en·home·be·da*	apaahoshe emempeeke *ah·bah·hose·he em·em·pee·ke*	gopher turtle food, gopher apple
42. meskolvpe *mis·kuh·luh·be*	'stapoochkeeke *stah·poch·kee·ke*	water oak
43. opv enhvfvtēhkv *o·puh en·huh·fuh·de·kuh*	oopaake oshtaape shapoke *o·pah·ke osh·tah·be sah·po·ke*	owl boots, mallow
44. opv 'mvhoswv *o·puh muh·hose·wuh*	oopaake embakshe *o·bah·ke em·buc·se*	owl threads, mallow
45. orko-latkv *oth·ko·lot·kuh*	olke *oth·ke*	flag pawpaw
46. passv *pas·shuh*	pashe *pa·she*	button snakeroot
47. poyvfekcv ekvhesse fvske *po·yuh·feek·chuh e·kuh·his·se fuhs·ke*	sholoopaale entokafashke *sho·lo·pah·the en·toe·kah·fahs·ke*	sharp hair spirits
48. poyvfekcv ensukcv-tvpekse *bo·yuh·feek·chuh en·suk·chuh·duh·beek·se*	sholoopaale enshokpachakfe *sho·loo·bah·the en·shoke·bah·chak·fe*	ghost bags, insect chrysalis
49. pvhe hvtke or hvtkuce *puh·he hut·ku·ce*	pahe hatkooche *pah·he hot·koo·che*	small white grass

Creek name	Mikasuki name	English common name
50. pvrko	batbe	grape
puth·go	*puth·be*	
51. pvto catuce	pakte keteschooche, shokhe-hatke hakchobe	red fungus
puh·do cha·due·che	*pak·de ke·tis·cho·che, shoke·he hut·ke hak·cho·be*	
52. roheleko	henle 'mashokche	mistletoe
thlo·he·le·ko	*hen·the mahs·hok·che*	
53. sakcometo	halpate mashoote	*alligator shader*, common button bush
sock·cho·me·do	*hul·pah·de mahs·hoe·de*	
54. 'stvlokpuce	tofoome	*hitchhiker*
sta·lok·po·gie	*toe·foo·me*	
55. sulecvpe	chowaane 'mochaape	wax myrtle
shoe·le·chuh·be	*cho·wah·ne mo·chah·be*	
56. svpeyv hvlwat	tofoome-chayhe	—
suh·be·yuh hul·wat	*to·foo·me chay·he*	
57. svpeyv-lopockuce	shapeye-peshkooshka	candy root
sa·be·yuh low·poch·ku·che	*sa·be·ye·pis·koosh·kah*	
58. svpeyv-rakko	shapeye-choobe	lantana
suh·be·yuh thak·ko	*suh·pe·ye cho·be*	
59. tartahkv	—	white ash
taht·tah·kuh		
60. tohome	ayekche-hoome	—
to·hoe·me	*ah·yeek·che ho·me*	
61. 'to-hvtkv	heekaape	Carolina ash
to·hut·kuh	*hee·kah·pe*	

#	Entry	Pronunciation	Alternate	Alt. pronunciation	English
62.	tolv	*tu·la*	toole	*tu·lee*	bay
63.	torkop-rakko	*toth·ko thack·ko*	etolpe-choobe	*e·toth·be cho·be*	water hemlock
64.	totkv cokhesse	*tot·kuh choke·his·se*	eete chooshke	*ee·te chosh·ge*	fire whiskers
65.	tvwv	*ta·wuh*	hekotaape	*he·ko·ta·pe*	winged sumac
66.	ue-heleswv	*we·he·lis·wa*	yahkaka-yekche	*yah·kaa·ka yeek·che*	lizard's tail
67.	vcenv	*uh·che·nuh*	achene	*a·che·ne*	cedar
68.	vktvpēhv	*uk·duh·be·huh*	akpolohlooche	*ak·bo·lo·lo·che*	*water floater*, floating hearts
69.	welanv	*we·la·nuh*	laykaape	*lay·kaah·be*	*stink plant*, wormseed
70.	wēso	*wee·so*	chahkane	*chah·kah·ne*	sassafras
71.	wotko elupe	*wot·ko e·loo·be*	shaawe loope	*shah·we loo·pee*	*raccoon or coon liver*
72.	wotko empvrko	*wot·ko em·puth·ko*	shaawe embalbe	*shah·we em·bawth·be*	*raccoon grape*
73.	yamēlikv	*yuh·me·lay·kuh*	ayekche-choobe	*ah·yeek·che cho·be*	*wolf's food*
74.	yvnvsv heleswv	*yuh·nuh·shvh he·les·wuh*	yanashe emayekche or pechekche emayekche	*pe·chek·che e·mah·yek·che*	*buffalo medicine*, black root

Appendix B. The Creek Alphabet

Letter	English sound	Creek word
A, a	awful, law	*halo, wakv*
C, c	juice, church	*cesse, cetto*
E, e	in, pin	*eco, este, wenketv*
Ē, ē	feed	*efēke, tuccēnen, hoktē*
F, f	fish	*fuswv, fo, tvlofv*
H, h	he, Bach	*hoktē, hvlpvtv*
I, i	lace	*yvpefikv, liketv*
K, k	get (gih)	*katcv, kute, hakkv*
L, l	lip	*lucv, tvlofv*
M, m	mouth	*mēkko, mahetv, emvhayv*
N, n	nose, sing	*nute, nokose, henkv*
O, o	hope	*opv, okeha, tvlofv*
P, p	pig, big, spot	*pokko, pose*
R, r	athlete	*raro, noricv*
S, s	sh, s, ts, z	*svmpv, sukhv*
T, t	stone (d)	*torwv, tolose*
U, u	wood	*fuswv*
V, v	but, luck	*vce, opv, svmpv*
W, w	we, wet	*ele-wesakv, hunvnwv*
Y, y	young	*yupo, yvnvsv, wvyo*

Diphthongs

au	house	*vhauke* (door)
ue	queen	*akhuervs* ("stand up!")

Appendix C. Alice's Genealogy

Alice Snow's mother's mother and others in her generation are not known except for her mother's sister, whose name was Lucy Tiger. In Seminole kinship terminology, the mother's mother's sisters would be called by the same name as the mother, indicating the extended kinship roles of matrilineal clan systems. Some of the dates that follow are approximate. All are arranged in birth order as remembered by Alice and other members of the community. Dates for some individuals were found in Jeff Bowen, *Seminole of Florida: Indian Census, 1930–1940 with Birth and Death Records, 1930–1938* (Signal Mountain, Tenn.: Mountain Press, 1997).

Alice Snow's father, Charlie Micco, and siblings in order of birth

Name	Year of birth	Clan	Spouse	Spouse's clan
Billy Tucker	1881	Panther	never married—Susie?	—
Charlie Micco	1892	Panther	Emma Maudey (Martin)	Bird
Sammy Jones	1894	Panther	Mercy (Missie Stick)	Bird
Oscar Hall	1896	Panther	To-chee or Cotner	Bird
Frank Shore	1900	Panther	Lottie Bowers (b. 1912)	Bird
Sally (Co-pic-cha-ho-lee)	1901	Panther	Sampson Snow	Bird
Sister (birth order not known)	—	Panther	—	—
Sister (birth order not known)	—	Panther	—	—

Alice Snow's mother, Emma Maudey (some say Martin), and siblings in order of birth

Name	Year of birth	Clan	Spouse	Spouse's clan
Charlie Snow	1896	Bird	never married	—
Sampson Snow	1896	Bird	Sally (Co-pic-cha-ho-lee)	Panther
Emma Maudey (Waswahkee)	1900	Bird	Charlie Micco	Panther

Children of Charlie Micco and Emma Maudey (Martin)

Name	Year of birth	Clan	Spouse	Spouse's clan
Little Charlie Micco	1916	Bird	Minnie (Mina) Osceola	Otter
Goby Micco	1919	Bird	Joe Henry Tiger	Panther
Leona Micco	1920	Bird	Jack Smith, Sr.	Panther
Cody Micco	1921	Bird	never married	—
Alice Louise Micco	1922	Bird	Bob Pearce Snow (b. 1920)	Panther
Jack Micco	1930	Bird	never married	—
Howard Micco	1934	Bird	Lois Johns	Panther

Children of Little Charlie Micco

Name	Clan	Spouse	Spouse's clan
Louise Cypress	Otter	Francis Osceola	Panther
Jerry Micco	Otter	(1) Joanne Osceola; (2) Carol Bowers	both Panther
Billy Micco	Otter	Mary Jo Jones	Panther
Jenny Mae Micco	Otter	Eddie Shore	Bird

Children of Goby Micco Tiger

Name	Clan	Spouse	Spouse's clan
Rosie Billie	Bird	(1) Johnny Buck; (2) Sammy Gopher	both Panther
Rufus Tiger	Bird	Martha Billie	Panther
Shirley Tiger	Bird	Gary Sampson	none
Amos Tiger	Bird	Lynell Whiddon	none

Children of Leona Micco Smith

Name	Clan	Spouse	Spouse's clan
Fred Smith	Bird	(1) Wanema Noel; (2) Ellen Click	no clan for either
Richard Smith	Bird	Elsie Johns	Panther
Nellie Smith	Bird	never married	—
Jack Smith, Jr.	Bird	Lois Johns	Panther
Oneva Smith	Bird	Buster Baxley	Panther
Roger Smith	Bird	Diane Snow	Panther
Linda Smith	Bird	Maxie Tommie	Deer
Paul Smith	Bird	died as child	—
Mahala Smith	Bird	John Madrigal	Panther

Children of Alice Micco Snow

Name	Clan	Spouse	Spouse's clan
Jennie Mae Snow	Bird	Jack Chalfant	none
Jim Snow	Bird	died as infant	—
Smawley Ollie Snow	Bird	Eli Holata	Alligator
Carolyn Snow (twin)	Bird	Gary Billie	Panther
Elbert Snow (twin)	Bird	(1) Laurie Comfort; (2) Judy Fortenberry	no clan for either
Salina Snow	Bird	John Dorgan	none

Appendix D. Plant Names for Mikasuki Speakers

◆◆◆◆◆◆◆◆◆◆◆◆◆◆◆◆◆◆◆

Common names in italics are literal translations.

Mikasuki name	Creek name	Common name	Botanical name
achene	vcenv	cedar	*Juniperus silicicola* (Small) Bailey
ahe-halbe	ahatkv	—	—
akpolohlooche	vktvpēhv	floating hearts, water floater	*Nymphoides aquaticum* (Walt.) Kunte
apaahoshe emempeeke	lucv-huehkv enhompetv	*gopher turtle food,* gopher apple	*Licania michauxii* Prance
ashayk-fomeeche	heno	red maple	*Acer rubrum* L.
ashoome-hatkooche	asvn-hvtkuce	British soldiers	—
atakle looche	vtakrv	dog fennel	*Eupatorium capillifolium* Lam. Small
atakle looche	atvkrv-lvste	dog fennel	—
ayekche-choobe	yamēlikv	*big medicine*	*Chrysobalanus oblongifolius* Michx.
ayekche-hatke	heles-hvtke	ginseng	*Panax quinquefolium* L.
ayekche-heele	heles-here	*good medicine,* downy milk pea	*Galactia volubilis* L. Britton
ayekche-hoome	tohome	*bitterwood*	—
balbe	pvrko	grape	*Vitis rufotomentosa* or *V. shuttleworthii* House
chahkane	wēso	sassafras	*Sassafras albidum* Nutt. Nees
chente ayekche	cetto enheleswv	*snake medicine,* clematis, leather flower	*Clematis baldwinii* Torri & Gray
chokfe empataake	cufe 'mvssv	*rabbit's bed,* panic grass	*Panicum zalapense* H.B.K. or *P. polycaulon* Nash
chokooche	culoswuce	*wild raisins,* little muscadine grape, scuppernong, little fox grape	*Cissus munsoniana* Simpson

chooye	cule	slash pine	*Pinus caribaea* Morelet
chooye enlepaatooche, chooye ebeele	cule emohlowakuce	pine tip	*Pinus caribaea* Morelet
eeche chaatehche	'coheceko	blind deer plant, goldenrod	*Solidago fistulosa* P. Miller or *S. canadensis* L.
eeche entohaane	'compvkanv	deer peaches	*Ximenia americana* L.
eeche hakchobe	eco hvcko vhakv	deer ears, sun-bonnet	*Chaptalia tomentosa* Vent.
eeche 'mahe	'comvhv	deer potato	*Liatris laxa*
emalopeeke looche	enkvtopokv-lvste	black-eyed Susan	*Rudbeckia hirta* L.
eptaape	hetotvpe	frost weed	*Verbesina virginica* L.
etolpe-choobe	torkop-rakko	water hemlock	*Cicuta maculata* L.
ewaashaake entapente	este-sumkat entvpentv	fern that grows in a cabbage palm	—
fayte emempeeke	efvkv-lanuce	golden threads, love vine	*Cassytha filiformis* Lauraceae
hache loopaape	helokhakv	strangler fig, rubber tree	*Ficus aurea* Nutt.
halpate choklaashe	hvlpvtv etolaswv vhakv	gator tongue, blue iris	*Crinum americanum* L.
halpate-mashoote	sakcometo	alligator shader, common button bush	*Cephalanthus occidentalis* L.
hamoohche loope entapente okecheske empakte	lakcv-cvmpv vloklopusat	lichen	—
hapooshekaaye-choobe	kvfockv	peppermint, penny royal sage	*Pycnothymus rigidus* Bart.
heekaape	'to-hvtkv, eto-hvtkv	Carolina ash	*Fraxinus caroliniana* Miller
hefepe-eele	hefepe or hefepe-nērkv	bottle gourd seeds	*Lagenaria siceraria* Mol.
hekotaape	tvwv	winged sumac	*Rhus copallina* L.
henle 'mashokche	roheleko	mistletoe	*Phoradendron serotinum* Raf. M.C. Johnston or *P. flavescens* Pursh Nutt.[2]

Mikasuki name	Creek name	Common name	Botanical name
heshke takhe	hesse-tvpehv	wide leaf	*Brassica oleracea* L.
kolotpahche ayekche	hoktvlkolowv enlocowv vhakuce	*old lady's paint pot, wide-open sore medicine*, hog food	*Ludwigia virgata* Michx.
kowaashe empataake	kowike entvlako	quail bean, partridge pea, or bird's foot trefoil	*Chamaecrista fasciculata* Michx. Greene C. *chamaecrista* L.
laykaape	welanv	stink plant, wormseed	*Chenopodium ambrosiodes* L.
okebakshe	akwanv	willow	*Salix amphibia*[3]
olke	orko-latkv	—	—
okecheske entapente	lakcv-cvmpv sohhontat	resurrection fern	*Polypodium polypodioides* L. Watt
olake	cafaknv	huckleberry, Darrow blueberry	*Vaccinium darrowii* Camp.
oopaake embakshe	opv 'mvhoswv	*owl threads*, mallow	Malvaceae
oopaake oshtaape shapoke	opv enhvfvtēhkv	*owl boots*, mallow	Malvaceae
pahe hatkooche	pvhe hvtke or hvtkuce	small white grass / sedge	*Pityopsis* sp.[4]
pakte keteschooche, shokhe-hatke hakchobe	pvto catuce	red fungus	—
pashe	passv	button snakeroot	*Eryngium yuccifolium* Michx.
pechekche emayeyce	yvnvsv heleswv	*blood medicine*, black root	*Pterocaulon pycnostachyum* Michx. Ellis
shaawe embatbe	wotko empvrko	raccoon grape	*Vitis cinerea*
shaawe loope	wotko elupe	raccoon or coon liver	*Stenandrium floridanum*
shachachapkooche	kvsvkakuce	rattle box	*Crotalaria pallida*
shachachapkooche	kvsvkakuce	rabbit bells	*Crotalaria pallida* or *C. rotundifolia* Walt. Gmel.
shapeye-choobe	svpeyv rakko	lantana	*Lantana camara* L.

shapeye-peshkooshka	svpeyv-lopockuce	candy root	—
sholoopaate enshokpachakfe	poyvfekcv-ensukcv tvpekse	*ghost bag or insect chrysalis*	—
sholoopaale entokafaske	poyvfekcv ekvhesse fvske	*sharp hair spirits*	—
showaane 'mochaape	sulecvpe	wax myrtle	*Myrica cerifera* L.
'stapoochkeeke	kvpopockv meskolvpe	water oak	*Quercus virginiana*
taapooche	coskelpv	elderberry	*Sambucus simpsoni*
tale sheetaaken	cvto ostet	*four smooth stones*	—
tofoome	estv lokpuce	beggar's lice	*Desmodium lineatum* or *D. supinam*
tofoome-chayhe	svpeyv hvlwat	—	—
toole	tolv	red bay	*Persea borbonia* L. Sprengel
wahole entayhe	halosvkatv entihv	*moccasin vine*, climbing hemp weed	*Mikania scandens* L. Willdenov
yaat-chayhe echooske	este hvlwat vhakuce	angel's hair, wild pine, *tall person hair*, ball moss	*Tillandsia setacea* SW or *Vittaria lineata* L.
yaat-hoboske emahe	este lopocke emeto	*where the little people live*	bundles of needles of *Pinus caribaea* Morelet
yahkaka-yekche	ue-heleswv	lizard's tail	*Saururus cernuus* L.
yakne chooshke	totkv cokhesse	*fire whiskers*	*Octoblepahrum albidum* Hedv.
yakne chooshke	ēkvnv cokhesse	ground whiskers, Beak rush	*Rhynchospora divergens* Chapm. Ex M.A. Curtis[5]
yanashe emayekche pechekche alahkahche emayekche	yvnvsv heleswv	black root, *buffalo medicine*	*Pterocaulon pycnostachyum* Michx. Ellis or *P. undulatum* Walt.
yooshnokaacheehche emayekche	lakcv-cvmpv tafvmpuce vhakusat sohhontusat	wild orchid, variety unknown	—

Notes

A Cherished Tradition

1. Literally, "two people pass each other."
2. H. Russell Bernard and Jesus Salinas Pedraza, *Native Ethnography: A Mexican Indian Describes His Culture* (Newbury Park, Calif.: Sage Publications, 1989).
3. In Oklahoma, the Creek language is referred to as Muskogee. Creek is used in Florida to describe the Florida dialect. Variations occur mostly in pronunciation and some words differ, but an Oklahoma speaker can understand the Florida speaker and vice versa. A Creek alphabet appears in Appendix B. Mikasuki is used here to refer to the Mikasuki language and its linguistic designation and is to be distinguished from the people who call themselves Miccosukee in Florida.
4. Jack Goody, "The Functions of Writing," *People and Plants Handbook: Sources for Applying Ethnobotany to Conservation and Community Development* 3 (1997): 23.
5. Ibid., 1 (editorial).

1. The Seminole People

1. William C. Sturtevant, "The Mikasuki Seminole: Medical Beliefs and Practices" (Ph.D. diss., Yale University, 1954), 68.
2. William C. Sturtevant, "Creek into Seminole," in *North American Indians in Historical Perspective*, ed. E. B. Leacock and N. O. Lurie (New York: Random House, 1971), 105.
3. James H. Howard (in collaboration with Willie Lena), *Oklahoma Seminoles: Medicine, Magic, and Religion* (Norman: University of Oklahoma Press, 1984); James W. Covington, *The Seminoles of Florida* (Gainesville: University Press of Florida, 1993).
4. Covington, *The Seminoles of Florida*, 72.
5. Harry A. Kersey, Jr., *An Assumption of Sovereignty: Social and Political Transformation among the Florida Seminoles, 1953–1979* (Lincoln: University of Nebraska Press, 1996).

6. In 1962, another group of Mikasuki-speaking individuals incorporated into a separate nation, the Miccosukee Tribe. Their residence and headquarters are along U.S. Highway 41 (the Tamiami Trail) in South Florida.

7. Seminole Tribe of Florida, "Tourism/Enterprises: What We Do" (http://www.semtribe.com/enterprises/), May 10, 2000.

8. Susan Enns Stans, "The Cultures of Drinking within a Native American Community" (Ph.D. diss., University of Florida, 1996).

9. Ibid.

10. Merwyn S. Garbarino, *Big Cypress: A Changing Seminole Community* (Prospect Heights, Ill.: Waveland Press, 1986 [1972]).

11. Little Bird was absorbed into Bird clan in the past.

12. R. T. King, "Clan Affiliation and Leadership among the Twentieth-Century Florida Indians, *Florida Historical Quarterly* 55 (1976): 135–52.

13. Stans, "Cultures of Drinking."

14. James O. Bushwell III, "Florida Seminole Religious Ritual: Resistance and Change" (Ph.D. diss., St. Louis University, 1972).

15. Covington, "The Seminoles of Florida," 211, 250.

16. Duane C. McBride and J. Bryan Page, "Final Report: Drug Abuse Demonstration Project of the Seminole Tribe of Florida" (Center for Social Research on Drug Abuse, University of Miami, 1978).

17. S. K. Joos, "Economic, Social, and Cultural Factors in the Analysis of Disease: Dietary Change and Diabetes Mellitus among the Florida Seminole Indians," in *Ethnic and Regional Foodways in the United States: The Performance of Group Identity,* ed. L. K. Brown and K. Mussell (Knoxville: University of Tennessee Press, 1984); D. N. Westfall and A. L. Rosenbloom, "Diabetes Mellitus among the Florida Seminoles," *HSMHA Health Reports* 86 (1971): 1037–41; Ruben H. Mayberry and Robert D. Lindeman, "A Survey of Chronic Disease and Diet in Seminole Indians in Oklahoma," *American Journal of Clinical Nutrition* 13, no. 3 (1963): 127–34.

18. Suzanne Davis, health educator, Department of Seminole Health, Hollywood, Florida, personal communication, 1998.

2. Seminole Traditional Medicine

1. Gary J. Martin, *Ethnobotany* (London: Chapman and Hall, 1995).

2. Quincy Spurlin, "Phytochemistry and Culture," *JCST* (September–October 1997): 23–28.

3. Peter B. Gallagher, *Seminole Tribune,* July 10, 1998, 1, 16.

4. William Sturtevant provides several of the songs in Creek/Muskogee translations in his unpublished dissertation, "The Mikasuki Seminole: Medical Beliefs and Practices" (Ph.D. diss., Yale University, 1954).

5. Ibid., 36.

6. The word *Busk,* another name for the Green Corn Dance, comes from the word (ibid., 104).

7. Ibid., 119–20.

8. Other plants are considered everything that is not medicine, or *heleswv tokoto* or *matokotos* (literally, "this is not it").

9. Ibid., 86.

10. Ibid., 110.

11. See "Alice's Seminole Rules of Life," this volume, 62.

12. Sturtevant calls it *ya:toposki*, which may be Mikasuki. This is one illness he ascribes to object intrusion. The little people shoot an arrow into the victim, causing illness. The remedy is extraction. Alice was unfamiliar with this concept (ibid., 216–17). In Jack B. Martin and Margaret Mckane Mauldin, *A Dictionary of Creek/Muskogee* (Lincoln: University of Nebraska Press, 2000), the authors describe little people as causing a person to get lost in the woods. Their work was done mostly in Oklahoma.

13. Greenlee acknowledges the relationship between dreams and sickness; however, he relates his observations to soul loss, which occurs when the person's ghost wanders at night via dreams and has such a pleasant time that it resists returning to the body in the morning. The resulting absence of the person's spirit causes the sickness. See Robert Greenlee, "Medicine of the Modern Florida Seminoles," *American Anthropologist* 46 (1944): 317–28.

14. Sturtevant concurs ("The Mikasuki Seminole," 122).

15. Daniel Moerman, "Physiology and Symbols: The Anthropological Implications of the Placebo Effect," in *The Anthropology of Medicine: From Culture to Method*, ed. Lola Romanucci-Ross, Daniel E. Moerman, and Laurence R. Tancredi (Westport, Conn.: Bergin and Garvey, 1997), 240.

3. Traditional Use of Plants

1. A. Douglas Kinghorn, "The Discovery of Drugs from Higher Plants," in *The Discovery of Natural Products with Therapeutic Potential*, ed. Vincent P. Gullo (Boston: Butterworth-Heineman, 1994), 97.

2. Ibid., 82.

3. Spurlin, "Phytochemistry and Culture," 26.

4. Kinghorn, "The Discovery of Drugs from Higher Plants," 83.

5. Arthur Osol, George E. Farrar, Jr., et al., *The Dispensatory of the United States of America*, 24th ed. (Philadelpia: Lippincott, 1947), in Sturtevant, "The Mikasuki Seminole," 242.

6. Daniel E. Moerman, *Native American Ethnobotany* (Portland, Ore.: Timber Press, 1999), 14.

7. *Hadassa Magazine*, December 1994, 40–41; see also Daniel Moerman, "Poisoned Apples and Honeysuckles: The Medicinal Plants of Native America," in *The Anthropology of Medicine: From Culture to Method*, ed. Romanucci-Ross, Moerman, and Tancredi, 61–70.

8. Alma R. Hutchens, *Indian Herbalogy of North America* (Boston: Shambhala, 1991), 138.

9. Spurlin, "Phytochemistry and Culture"; Moerman, *Native American Ethnobotany*; Moerman, "Poisoned Apples and Honeysuckles."

10. Moerman, *Native American Ethnobotany*, 14.

11. Michelle M. Alexander and J. Anthony Parades, "Possible Efficacy of a Creek Folk Medicine through Skin Absorption: An Object Lesson in Ethnopharmacology," *Current Anthropology* 39 (August–October 1998): 545–49.

12. Christopher Hallowell, "The Plant Hunter," *Time* (Fall 1997): 17–21.

13. Wilhelmina F. Greene and Hugo L. Blomquist, *Flowers of the South* (Chapel Hill: University of North Carolina Press), 83.

14. Hutchens, *Indian Herbalogy*, 140.

15. Literally, "herbs to collect."

16. Frances Densmore, *How Indians Use Wild Plants for Food, Medicine, and Crafts* (New York: Dover Publications, 1974).

17. Hutchens, *Indian Herbalogy*.

18. Called free listing in Gary J. Martin, *Ethnobotany* (London: Chapman and Hall, 1995), and H. Russell Bernard, *Research Methods in Anthropology* (Thousand Oaks, Calif.: Sage Publications, 1994).

19. Greene and Blomquist, *Flowers of the South*, 84.

20. Charles Hudson, *The South Eastern Indians* (Knoxville: University of Tennessee Press, 1976).

21. Densmore, *How Indians Use Wild Plants*, 302, 304–5.

22. Genus (plural genera) refers to the first name in the Linnean classification system (example: *Persea borbonia*). The binomial or two-name system uses genera to classify different species of plants that have certain properties in common.

4. Alice's Story: "When I Was Coming Up . . ."

1. A hanging baby cradle made by sewing a blanket between two ropes that are tied parallel to each other.

2. "Little baby, come on. Little baby, come on."

3. Jim died in infancy.

4. To get the children to behave, Alice always wore a large safety pin at the hem of her shirt when she was working at the Head Start program. Although she never used the pin, she would tell the children that when they misbehaved, they would get scratched and change their conduct. At a rodeo once, one of the little children came up to ask to see the pin. Alice turned over the hem of the shirt to show him. He whooped, "Oooooh" and hurried away. He had wanted to show his little friend the fearsome thing. Whippings and scratching are no longer used as methods of punishment for the children, but the thought of the punishment lingers in the culture. The scratchings performed at the Green Corn Dance today are symbolic of initiation

into manhood and purification, rather than disciplinary measures for cultural transgressions. Men wear their old and new scars from the corn dance proudly.

7. Plant Identification Chart for Creek Speakers

1. English names in italics are literal translations from the Creek or Mikasuki.

2. *S. amphibia* is scarce in the area so *S. carolinia* is used.

3. Turkeys eat the berries.

4. A Cyperaceae (sedge family) Sturtevant identifies as *Eleocharis caribaea* Rothb.

5. Caution: fresh root is poisonous.

6. Sturtevant cites orko as custard apple, but the herb Alice calls orko is not that but a pawpaw.

7. Perhaps both are *P. graminifolia* Michx. Nutt., but we need the flowers to make sure neither one is *Chrysopsis*.

8. Caution: berries are poisonous.

9. Caution: poisonous.

Appendix D. Plant Names for Mikasuki Speakers

1. Caution: fresh flag root is poisonous.

2. Caution: berries are poisonous.

3. *Salix amphibia* is scarce in the area so *S. carolinia* is used.

4. Perhaps both are *P. graminifolia* Michx. Nutt., but we need the flowers to make sure neither one is *Chrysopis*.

5. A Cyperaceae (sedge family) Sturtevant identifies as *Eleocharis caribaea* Rothb.

Subject Index

Note: Numbers in italics refer to photographs.

observation and Indian medicine, 24
Oklahoma, 14, 43, 61
"on the wagon" medicine, xii, 24–25, 26, 86–88, color plate 16
oral tradition, 2
Osceola, 14
Osceola, Frances, *18*
Osceola, Onnie, *18*
owl sickness, color plate 32

pain, treatment of, 25–26, 69–70, 76
Panther clan, 19, 27
Parades, Anthony, 36–37
patient: role of, 25; tailoring amount of medicine to, 7
placebo effect, 33
plants: commonly used, 41–43; ethnobotany and, 34; for healing, 34–36; identification chart of, 96–99; known by Alice Snow, 104–9; poisonous, 36; range of, 42–43; supplies of, 37–38; tools for gathering, *38*. *See also* herb collection; index of plants
population of Brighton Reservation, 17
possessions of dead person, 90
pregnancy, protection of baby during, 82–83

Radin, Paul, 4
religion, 19–20, 60. *See also* Green Corn Dance
restrictions: after birth, 54–58; hospitals and, 28; "on the wagon" medicine, 26

salicylates, natural, 36
Salinas Pedraza, Jesus, 4
scratching, 126–27n.4
Second Seminole War, 14
Seminole, meaning of, 13
Seminole medicine: elements of, 25; importance of, 28; practice of, xi, 2, 24–25
Seminole people: clans of, 16, 18–19, 21; and dress contest, *18, 55*; education of, 20–21; health concerns of, 28–29; history of, 13–15; language of, 4–6, 8–9, 13–14, 15–16; reservations for, 15; Tribe, incorporation of, 15–16; view of members of, 23. *See also* Brighton Reservation
Seminole Rules of Life, 62

shortness of breath, treatment of, 73
sleep, treatment of, 75–76, 78–79, color plate 32
Smith, Fred, *52*, 114
Smith, Jack, Jr., xi–xiii, 3, *54*, 114
Smith, Leona Micco: with Alice, *57*; children of, 114; family of, 44, *54*; herbs and, xv, 52; work of, xi–xii
Smith, Lois Johns, xii–xiii, 114
Smith, Nellie, *54*, 114
Snow, Alice: award to, *22*; bicultural, 4; birth of, 44; as board representative, 49; at Brighton Indian Day School, *47, 48*; and Brighton Reservation, 16–17; children of, *54, 56, 58*, 115; counting game, *46*; criticism of, 1–2; description of, 1; dreams of, 31–32; and dress contest, *18*; early life of, 44–45, *45, 46, 47, 50*; on education, 49; education of, 47–49; evolution of book by, 3–4; family of, 44, *61*; gathering tools of, *38*; genealogy of, 113–15; herb collection experiences of, 6–8, *39, 40, 41*, 51–52, 59–60; and hunting, 49–50; independence of, 62–63; as Indian doctor, 58; as interpreter, 47, 49; and knee surgery treatment, 25–26; knowledge of, xi; languages of, 47, 49, 52; marriage of, 52–53; mission of, 8–9; petition by, 21–23; plants known by, 104–9; religion of, 60–61; Seminole Rules of Life by, 62; with sister, *57*; teaching by, xiii–xiv; travels of, 61–62; work of, xi–xiii, 47, 49, 63
Snow, Bob, 52–53, 114
Snow, Carolyn, 54, *58*, 115
Snow, Elbert, xii, xiii–xiv, 54, *58*, 115
Snow, Jenny, 54, 115
Snow, Smawley, 54, *56*, 115
social structure of Brighton Reservation, 18–19
songs of Indian doctor: for death medicine, 60; for "fixing" medicine, 7; learning of, 7–8, 27; purpose of, xv, 2; role of, 25; "spiritual transmission" and, 37
soul loss, 125n. 13
Southern Baptist religion, 20, 60
speeding heart, treatment of, 73–74
"spiritual transmission," 37

stone, treatment with, 86, 87
stroke medicine, 30–31, 37, 40–41, 72
Sturtevant, William, 24, 28, 42
surgery, treatment after, 25–26, 67–68

teaching: public education and, 8–9; traditional styles of, 1–2, 7–8, 51–52
Third Seminole War, 14, 44
Thomas, Michelle, 3
Tiger, Goby Micco, 44, 114
Tiger, Mary, 52
Tiger, Rufus, 54, 114
transdermal application, 36–37
treatments: after surgery, 25–26, 67–68; for alcohol abuse, xii, 24–25, 26, 86–88, color plate 16; for arthritis, 36; "as told to" method and, 5; for baby, 35, 54–58, 83–86; for blackouts or shortness of breath, 73; body washes, 36–37; categories of, 29–33; cold/cool medicine, 33, 67–68; for crying baby, 35; death medicine, 88–90, color plates 4, 17; for dreams and sleep, 26, 31–32, 75–76, 78–79, color plate 32; for ear, 71; for fear of walking after long illness, 74–75; gifts in exchange for, 26, 27–28; for high blood pressure, color plate 16; hysterectomy, 68–69; length of time for, 7; for loss of husband or wife, 90–92; for menstrual period, 82; for miscarriage, 81–82; mixed medicine, 77; for monkey sickness, 30, 33, 80; for owl sickness, color plate 32; for pain, 25–26, 69–70, 76; during pregnancy (to protect baby), 82–83; restrictions and, 26, 28; for sleeping all the time, 75–76; for speeding heart, 73–74; stroke medicine, 30–31, 37, 40–41, 72; "white people" and, 7, 37; for worm sickness, 34–35
Treaty of Moultrie Creek, 14

walking, fear of after long illness, 74–75
Western medicine, 2, 28, 35
white grits (osafke hvtke), 76, 84, 85, 91
"white people," treatments and, 7, 37
wife, loss of, 90–92
women in Seminole Tribe, 16, 29, 58
worm sickness, 34–35
writing, functions of, 5

Index of Plants

Alice Snow is an elder of the Seminole Tribe of Florida. She works as a liaison between Seminole traditional doctors and the Seminole people. She lives at Brighton Reservation, near Okeechobee, not far from where she was born. Alice is active in the First Indian Baptist Church and the senior program in her community. In the past she served as Brighton Board Representative, one of the tribe's governing bodies. She also takes classes at Florida Gulf Coast University.

Susan Stans is an assistant professor of anthropology at Florida Gulf Coast University. While she was working toward a Ph.D. in anthropology from the University of Florida, she served a twenty-month dissertation residency at the Brighton Reservation, where she lived with Alice Snow. Her academic appointment is partially funded by a grant from the Seminole Tribe of Florida, which allows her to teach half-time and serve half-time as mentor to Seminole students and as university liaison to the Seminole education department. She also conducts a summer school program at the reservation.

This book is the first for each author.